A GUIDE FOR

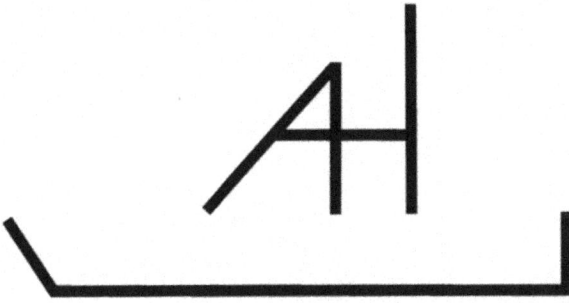

AGING HEROES

30 Days to Owning the Second Half of Life

Randolph Harrison, MEd.
with Erica Schwarting

Black Rose Writing | Texas

First printing

ISBN: 978-1-68513-238-5
PUBLISHED BY BLACK ROSE WRITING
www.blackrosewriting.com

Printed in the United States of America
Suggested Retail Price (SRP) $19.95

A Guide for Aging Heroes is printed in Sabon

*As a planet-friendly publisher, Black Rose Writing does its best to eliminate unnecessary waste to reduce paper usage and energy costs, while never compromising the reading experience. As a result, the final word count vs. page count may not meet common expectations.

PRAISE FOR
A GUIDE FOR

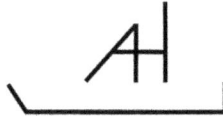

AH

AGING HEROES

"...in grasping the significance of this work, we are led almost inevitably to realize that this is the approach that we should adopt to access a fulfilling and satisfying future. A well–written and inspiring text, filled with mature insights garnered from a lifetime of experience."
–Lois Henderson for *Readers' Favorite*

"This book is beyond life–changing. It allowed me to take a look at my life and make the necessary changes. Highly recommend this to all who are looking to better themselves and their lives. If you take this book seriously and put in the work, you will become an Aging Hero."
–Dog–Eared Reviews

"When applied correctly, you will find that the strategies provided will break down the barriers created by past childhood and relationship trauma. Discover the benefits of living a joyful life, investing in experiences, and becoming an Aging Hero."
–Luwi Nyakansaila for *Readers' Favorite*

"...the transformative power of this book... will lead you on a spiritual journey and help you overcome life's challenges with renewed confidence, ease, and grace."
–Thomas Anderson, Editor In Chief for *Literary Titan*

For Lainey, Harry, and Tallas

ACKNOWLEDGMENTS

My most profound appreciation goes to my wife and co-creator, Erica Schwarting, who collaborated on every chapter, and without whom, I could never have written this book. I am indebted to our children, Lainey Harrison, Harry Harrison, and Tallas Lineberger, who constantly inspire me to be a better person. Gratitude to my sister Leanne Tyson who is a never-ending source of love and support. My deepest thanks to Reagan Rothe and the expert staff at Black Rose Writing for bringing this project to fruition. Thanks to everyone who has ever had a meaningful conversation with Erica or me about an important topic. And heartfelt appreciation to all of you aging heroes out there who inspired this work.

A GUIDE FOR

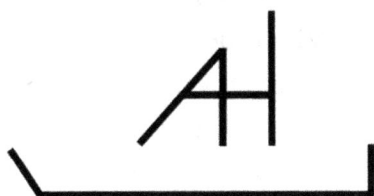

AGING HEROES

PREFACE

The concept of *aging heroes* fermented for several years before it was fully formed. My beautiful wife, Erica, and I had an ongoing conversation about defining what it means to be *cool*. We started by trying to determine if there is anything that is always *cool*, a universal litmus. I suggested blues music, motorcycles, and rebellion. Erica disagreed with all three. She considers jazz music cooler than blues, and she said motorcycles and rebellion both exist on a continuum from infantile to cool. When the rubber hit the road, we could not come up with a single thing that was universally cool. Any and every style of music, clothing, or mode of transportation had the potential to be cool. Likewise, any hobby or pastime had that same potential. We decided that *cool* must be defined by each individual and born of authenticity. People who dare to be their authentic selves have the privilege of determining what is cool. Conversely, inauthentic conformists have no access to cool.

As people move through middle and old age, they seem to have two potential trajectories. They either double down on complying with societal norms and calcify into mediocre lives or create their own paths and, like the velveteen rabbit, become more and more real. Folks who take this second course are what we call *aging heroes*. Each hero's life is an eccentric work of art molded by thought, word, and deed. While very different from one another, aging heroes have a few things in common. They all have courage, nobility of character, concern for others, curiosity, self-awareness, a sense of adventure, and a commitment to personal development. For *aging heroes*, life becomes richer, fuller, and more fun as they grow older. Aging heroes are cool!

The world is speckled with aging heroes. Erica and I are proud to count ourselves among them. We found each other late in life after many failed relationships. Neither of us has ever lived on more than a middle-class income. We are an interracial couple living in the foothills of Western North Carolina, and we're on the back end of middle age. However, despite it all, we are living extraordinary lives that get better and better! We have been on safari in Tanzania and explored the jungles of Panama. We sponsored multiple charity events at home and abroad. We have friends all over the world. We surf, sail, study, backpack, run, read, swim, sing, play, contribute, write, travel, and follow our hearts wherever they lead us. I can't imagine a more satisfying existence!

So many good people are stuck on the hamster wheel of societal expectations doing everything they are supposed to but still feeling unfulfilled. Creating emotional prosperity requires making attitude shifts and acquiring skills across all of life's domains. Becoming aging heroes has been a learning process for Erica and me. We are not unique. Anyone can make the change. This book represents our offer to share the love. Here's to living your best life now!

CONTENTS

INTRODUCTION

"Twenty years from now you will be more disappointed by things you didn't do than by the ones you did do. So throw off the bowlines. Sail away from the safe harbor. Catch the trade winds in your sails. Explore. Dream. Discover."[i]

~ H. Jackson Brown Jr.

The media's depictions of people going through the second half of life are overwhelmingly negative. We are characterized as less attractive, less bright, less able-bodied, and ultimately less relevant than our younger counterparts. Consider how often aging is associated with being slow, sickly, frail, forgetful, or needy. Such stereotypes tend to burrow into our unconscious minds and become self-fulfilling prophecies. Fortunately, with introspection and conscious effort, we can root out destructive myths and embrace the reality that growing older can be a terrific, life-affirming adventure!

The difference between an aging hero and the average person can be captured in one word, courage. Courage defines heroes. Aging heroes have the mettle to rail against the confines of conventional attitudes. We embrace opportunities to create meaning in our lives and to improve the lives of others. Prisoners of modern social constructs are unaware that the key to freedom is always within reach. That key is the courage to step out of their assigned roles and live authentically. In a world often governed by fear and negativity, aging heroes gaze on the future with confidence, enthusiasm, and wonder.

Aging Heroes is a lifestyle. Adopt it as you navigate the waters of middle and late adulthood. You express your lifestyle in everything you do. Your work, habits, attitudes, choices, how you interact with others, and what you do for fun are all expressions of your lifestyle. As an aging hero, these expressions fall into a harmonious rhythm flowing from your truest, most authentic self. Fair warning, though, this voyage is not for everyone. Older does not always mean wiser. It isn't difficult to find people of all ages stuck in unhealthy patterns and unwilling to do anything about it. Some live with their eyes closed, never recognizing the harm they cause or the wonderful opportunities they waste. They lack the courage, insight, and maturity to be aging heroes. All aging heroes are committed to moving beyond the status quo. The number one regret of the dying is that they did not live lives true to themselves but instead tried to conform to what others expected of them.[ii] Aging heroes refuse to be defined by others. We create lives distinguished by self-discovery, adventure, service, and personal growth.

The old saying, "the whole is more than the sum of its parts," is fundamental to the Aging Heroes' credo. Think of a delicious chocolate cake. The cake is more than the eggs, flour, sugar, cocoa, and butter used to make it. With the help of the baker, the cake has emerged from these ingredients as something altogether different. You are, likewise, more than your physical body, more than your thoughts, more than your experiences, and more than your relationships. You emerge from all of these a singular and ever-transforming entity.

The components that create you are dynamic. That is, they are constantly interacting with each other. These interactions result in the change and progress you experience in your life. Likewise, you are a dynamic component of a greater system. Your interactions with the environment around you ultimately influence change and progress in the world! Desmond Tutu said, "Do your little bit of good where you are. It's those little bits of good put together that overwhelm the world."[iii]

Everything is interconnected. The people, things, and events in your life affect you as you, in turn, affect them. In my family, we talk about how moods can be contagious. If one person in our house is irritable, the rest of us may soon follow suit. Every action you take in life creates a ripple in the fabric of the whole. The action may cause a tiny ripple, as when someone does you a small kindness, and you pay it forward to others. Or, it may cause a big ripple that impacts history, such as when Rosa Parks chose to sit in the front of the bus.

From you, me, Erica (my beautiful wife/co-creator), and others like us emerges Aging Heroes. We are works in progress, ever-improving. As we take on the challenges of this quest, we are also creating positive ripples that affect the world around us. By living our best lives, we ignite that passion in others.

A Guide for Aging Heroes provides tools that can help you create a vibrant existence at any age. All recommendations relating to wellness are supported by research.

CASTING OFF

"The cure for everything is salt water: sweat, tears, or the sea."[iv]
~ Isak Dinesen

Every ocean passage begins with some planning. You must set a course, stow away provisions, inspect your equipment, and garner some expertise before setting sail. The journey of an aging hero also requires preparation. You have to outfit yourself with patience and optimism. You must plan to be bold in examining yourself, decisive in choosing your direction in life, and tenacious in your pursuit of change. Radical transformation is possible.

START A NOTEBOOK

Keep a notebook and a pencil or pen handy as you read the chapters. Taking occasional notes and following through on suggested activities can help you get the most from *A Guide for Aging Heroes*.

If you have a significant other, consider working through the process together. If you are not currently in a relationship, you may want to work through the book with anyone close to you. Erica and I covered each chapter and completed the notebook activities together. We had a good time, and it gave us insights into ourselves and each other.

DAY 1: DAY ONE OR ONE DAY

"You don't have to be great to start, but you have to start to be great."[v]
~ Zig Ziglar

Which will you choose today, *day one*, or *one day*? Will today be the day you really begin to live, or will you put it off again? I lived much of the first half of my life in endless procrastination. *"One day*, I will get in shape. *One day* I will travel. *One day* I will write a book."

There is a Buddhist parable about an elderly monk doing heavy labor in the hot sun without a hat. A traveler noticed the old man and felt sorry for him.

"Why not have one of the younger monks do that?" asked the traveler.

"Because that would not be me," answered the old monk.

"Why not at least wait until later in the day when the sun is not so hot?" proposed the traveler.

"Because that would not be now," smiled the monk.

The old monk understood that only he could live his life and that the only time to live it was in the present moment. Imagine your best life. What does it look like? How close are you to living that life? What steps will you need to take to get there? What can you do right now to move in that direction?

My wife, Erica, tends to live in the now, but it took a significant health crisis to wake me up and choose *day one* instead of yet another *one day*. A few years ago, I was diagnosed with COPD. It is a chronic, progressive, incurable lung disease. I have always been into fitness and had every intention of retiring with Erica on a boat and sailing the seven seas. This diagnosis was a punch in the gut. I freaked out.

COPD means gradually suffocating to death. In the end stages, people with this condition struggle for every breath and have difficulty doing simple activities like walking and getting dressed.

The comfortable fantasy that I would die at 96 having some crazy adventure went right out the window. I became profoundly depressed and threw in the towel. I drank heavily and obsessed with the prospect of dying for months. It was also, of course, a challenging time for Erica. Not only did she have to deal with her concerns over my physical health, but she also had to manage a husband who was mentally falling to pieces. Eventually, with her support, I took back control of my life. I have outlined many of the strategies I used to do so in this book. You may not have experienced walking out of your doctor's office with life-altering health news, but there is a good chance, at some point, you will. How will you deal with it?

Emily Dickinson said, "That it will never come again is what makes life so sweet."[vi] My dad died from an aortic aneurysm at age 69. His doctor compared it to being struck by lightning. Not a terrible way to check out. He was never decrepit, never senile. He had tackled a purse snatcher six months before his death and spent the morning driving a transfer truck the day he died. I often wonder how his final days might have been different if Daddy had known that the last sunset he saw would be the last sunset he would ever see and the last time he kissed my mother would be the last time he would ever kiss her. Wouldn't he have cherished those experiences and made himself fully present for them?

I think the gift of my diagnosis was an opportunity to re-prioritize. A chance to tune in to the people I love and invest myself in truly meaningful efforts. I have no interest in quietly fading away. I will charge into the future with passion and creativity. I will engage the remaining stages of my life on my terms and will not allow a diagnosis to spill wind from my sails.

The great social psychologist, Erik Erikson, described two stages in the second half of life. Each stage has two possible outcomes, one positive and one negative.

The potential outcomes in middle age are either *generativity* or *stagnation*.[vii] The term *generativity* comes from the word *generous*. By middle age, many people have achieved a certain level of stability. Healthy adults at this stage of life are compelled to give back. They may invest themselves in raising well-adjusted children, nurturing a loving relationship with a significant other, or getting involved in their communities by volunteering, making donations, or joining a charity organization, the PTA, or an activist group. Generativity includes caring for future generations and all people, not just friends, family, and self.

Giving is qualitatively more rewarding than receiving.[viii] Think of how uncomfortable it is to ask a stranger for a jump when your car battery dies in a parking lot. If someone helps you, you feel grateful and probably a little embarrassed. Now consider what it is like to be on the giving end in that scenario. When you can give a stranger a jump because *they* have a dead battery, you are the hero of the story, and it feels wonderful. The benefits of altruism, kindness for its own sake, include a release of positive neurochemicals called endorphins.[ix] The same chemicals are released during the "runner's high." Altruism gives you a sense of fulfillment and gratitude for your own circumstances. Helping others puts your problems in perspective and makes you physically healthier by reducing stress! Generativity is the hallmark of success in mid-life.

The potential unsuccessful outcome in midlife is *stagnation*. Life becomes stale for stagnated folks causing them to be increasingly resentful, jealous, and self-serving. These people continuously try to fill the void in their lives with material gain. Snobs and braggarts fall into this category. Think of Ebenezer Scrooge, the haughty lady at the country club, or the self-aggrandizing billionaire. Stagnated people often have everything society says should make them happy, but they are still empty. They want more.[x] Their lives lack genuine purpose, and no amount of money or power can relieve their need. What's worse is they pass on this spiritual vacuum to their children, who suffer high rates of anxiety, depression, and substance abuse.[xi] Stagnated individuals typify selfishness.

How are you measuring up? Are you involved and engaged in making the world a better place, or are you mainly just looking out for yourself and the people close to you? Most social animals will help members of their group. A wolf will instinctively help members of its own pack but would be unlikely to show prosocial behavior toward wolves from other packs. "Looking out for your own" is an innate animal behavior. Emotionally mature humans can do more. Humans can express their regard to people and things outside their social groups. This represents one of the noblest characteristics a human being can develop.

Regardless of age, it is never too late to recalibrate your priorities. If you feel stagnated, make this *day one* and do something to foster generativity. Any random act of kindness will be a foot placed on the right path. You will be amazed at how a simple act of kindness for its own sake affects your self-satisfaction and shifts perceptions about your fellow human beings.

The final stage of life, old age, is marked by either integrity or despair.[xii] If successful, you look backward and forward with satisfaction that you have lived and are living your best life. You operate according to your own rules and not the expectations of others. You appreciate the virtue and wisdom you have gained. This is integrity. When you have lived with integrity, you feel whole and complete. Integrity defines success in the final stage of life.

Unsuccessful people in the last chapter of life experience despair.[xiii] Their lives are riddled with guilt, regret, and hopelessness. They cry, "Why me? My life is over, and what did it all mean? I never became the person I wanted to be. I never made a difference. It isn't fair!"

Do you have a sense of wholeness? Are you at peace with how you live and have lived? If not, what can you do right now to change course?

I love the idea of the Aging Hero. As Erica and I developed the concept, we had people we know in mind. They are people who are in love with being alive. They contribute. They create. They connect. They make a difference. They are living representations of generativity and integrity. The impermanence of life is a guidepost that provides direction and motivation to live authentically. I no longer have time to waste wishing my life away, and neither do you.

Fyodor Dostoevsky said, "Taking a new step, uttering a new word, is what people fear most."[xiv] People fear getting started. Do not wait to *feel* motivated. Start now, regardless of your feelings. Motivation is born of momentum, and momentum doesn't build while you wait for the perfect mood to strike you. Life is happening while you wait! Joy and self-worth come from living the life you want and not from dreaming about that life. *One day* is an illusion. A bottomless abyss of delayed fulfillment. Leave your mark on this world. Do good deeds. Live the life you were meant to live. *Day one* begins now! Take up the challenge and be an example for others.

NOTEBOOK ACTIVITY: THIS IS DAY ONE

In your notebook, write down this date. This is your Day One. Tomorrow may also be Day One. If needed, you can have a long series of days that are Day One until it sticks. The only way to fail at this is to stop trying. Write out your intention to start living your best life now. How can you make generativity and integrity the outcomes in your life? What obstacles might get in the way of your success? List a few strategies you might use to overcome those barriers as they arise.

DAY 2: TRANSFORM

"Someone I loved once gave me a box full of darkness. It took me years to understand that this, too, was a gift"[xv]
~ Mary Oliver

Developing an Aging Heroes lifestyle is a transformative process that reshapes the ordinary into the extraordinary. Erica and I are fascinated by the notions of transformation and rebirth. Rebirth is a metaphor that runs deep in the ancestral memories of human beings. In the Christian religion, Easter is celebrated in spring, signifying Christ's transformation from death to life. Spring itself is a symbol of rebirth. In winter, plants go dormant and appear dead. Many animals hibernate. When spring arrives, nature comes alive again. Taoism, Hinduism, and Buddhism capture rebirth with the concept of reincarnation. Humans have endless opportunities to "get life right" by being reborn into different forms. Pagan religions express the idea of renewal in their celebration of the winter solstice or Yule. The winter solstice is the shortest day of the year, after which the days grow longer. The sun's return is observed by lighting candles and yule logs and decorating homes with holly and evergreens. All are symbols of transformation from dark to light and from death to life.

The ancient Greeks and Egyptians have stories about a mythical bird called the *phoenix* that symbolizes the sun and rebirth. The phoenix was a grand and beautiful creature with a lifespan of hundreds of years. But only one phoenix at a time was ever in existence. When it died, the phoenix would be consumed in flames. A new phoenix would then rise from its predecessor's ashes even greater than before. Each aging hero is a phoenix. We are consumed by the flames of trauma, heartbreak, and hardship, and then we rise from the ashes, stronger and wiser than before.

I once spoke with a very old woman named Aileen, who described this process in a way that moved me. She said, "When I was young, I was anxious and fragile. A gentle breeze could blow me over. Then, I lived through poverty, the Great Depression, two world wars, and the deaths of so many people I loved. Now, I can stand tall in a hurricane, and it is almost time for me to leave." Aileen was a phoenix.

Erica grew up as a minority to minorities. One of her birth parents was white, the other black. As an infant, she was adopted by white parents from New York and raised by them in Western North Carolina. With an adopted family from New York, many things about Erica were very different from those in her community. Her dialect, social and political views, and diet were unlike those in her North Carolina circle. Erica was too black for white people and too white for black people. Southern Appalachia is a hard place to grow up if you are African American, but it is an impossible place if you are a person of color who other people of color shun. Erica is a quiet person, and she describes feeling invisible in school. To a large degree, she lived a life of solitude.

The fires of isolation and rejection incinerated Erica, but she emerged as one of the strongest, most caring people I have ever known. She is deeply involved in charity work and is always willing to pitch in when people need help. In her everyday life, she gives and gives and gives. She is skilled at deflecting the daily slights that people from all minority groups have to manage. Her challenges have given her an inner strength that floors me.

I am a reasonably attractive, reasonably intelligent, white, middle-class male raised in the Southeastern U.S. When it comes to being born into privilege, I pretty much hit the jackpot for everything but wealth. Considering these circumstances, I might easily have become a selfish, hard-hearted asshole. Finding people with my background who turned out like that is not difficult. However, I also have a mood disorder called major depression. I've endured depressive episodes that I would not wish on my worst enemy.

Ultimately though, I am grateful for the gifts depression has provided. Depression has given me not only depths of emotion that are inaccessible to people without the condition but also insight into the suffering of others. Depression has endowed me with empathy. Empathy is not sympathy. For kind people, compassion is easy. Feeling sorry for folks who are suffering comes naturally to caring people. Empathy requires effort. Empathy demands mentally putting yourself in another person's place and trying to understand the world from their point of view. Practicing empathy for people you don't like can be uncomfortable. You must put your ego on the back burner to pull it off. Charles M. Blow said, "One does not have to operate with great malice to do great harm. The absence of empathy and understanding is enough."[xvi] Well-developed empathy skills are uncommon. Cultivating genuine empathy should be on everyone's to-do list.

As a child, I was a low achiever with terrible self-esteem. I was small, insecure, and constantly bullied. I was the last one picked for any team sport and was regularly ridiculed and humiliated. In the schoolyard pecking order, I was at the very bottom. Like many victims of bullies, I had a rich fantasy life where I was strong and brave. In my dreams, the bullies all met with a reckoning, and I was the hero.

The themes of my imaginary play always centered on a downtrodden underdog who would overcome insurmountable odds or die trying. I loved imagining the old athlete past his prime continuing to compete valiantly against younger and stronger opponents. Whenever I went to the beach, I would build sandcastles with multiple moats and walls to protect them from the incoming tide. As the waves came in, I would struggle in vain to reinforce the walls knowing that, ultimately, the sea would always win. In retrospect, the process was an excellent metaphor for life. Every life ends in the same tragedy with no way to escape the fate of dying. What matters is how you work to meet life's challenges until that tide washes you away.

In childhood, I was courageous in my fantasies and timid in life. Except for a handful of cousins who were my best friends growing up, I avoided other kids. I was terrified of public attention and stayed away from crowds at all costs. It took me years to come to terms with the torment I went through as a kid. Education, self-reflection, and more than a few fistfights eventually helped me come out on the other side.

I was swallowed by the fires of depression and childhood bullying, but from those ashes emerged an empathetic advocate for disadvantaged people. I give a pass to the child bullies who tortured me. In their families, they were probably victims themselves. Conversely, I hold adult bullies accountable. Erica and I actively campaign against injustice in all its miserable forms. Bigotry, racism, homophobia, and antisemitism are just alternative names for bullying. We live in an age that glorifies bullies. Financially successful bullies are admired as role models. Concern for the welfare of less fortunate people is derided as a sign of weakness and naivety. Bullies have even affected our language. One expression, "political correctness," has enhanced the smug disregard bullies feel for marginalized groups. The term "politically correct" has replaced what we used to call "good manners."

I think the intellectual, emotional, and physical development Erica and I enjoy now can be traced to experiences of feeling helpless and alone as children. I wonder what lackluster lives we might have accepted if we hadn't gone through that suffering. Could we have become weak-minded bullies ourselves?

There are undoubtedly sad people who are beaten down by life and never recover. Why are traumatic experiences transformative for some people and not for others? Aside from legitimate mental health issues, I think the difference is one's understanding of freedom and responsibility. We are each thrown into life under circumstances over which we have no control.[xvii] Some of us land in wealth and opportunity, others in poverty and persecution. That part of life is a crapshoot, and nothing about it is fair. What we choose to do with those circumstances is where responsibility becomes the determining factor.

A child whose life is miserable because she is growing up in difficult circumstances is pretty powerless to change her situation. An adult whose life is miserable because she grew up in difficult circumstances as a kid has not only the freedom but also the responsibility to change it.[xviii] This is not to say that everyone has the life skills to overcome such a challenge. Sometimes seeking and accepting help from others is a necessary part of the process. Ultimately, the power and the responsibility for initiating change lie with the individual. People who take responsibility for their lives in the present, regardless of the cards they have been dealt, are phoenixes.

NOTEBOOK ACTIVITY: THE FLAMES IN YOUR LIFE

List the events that have created the fire for your transformation. Take a minute to appreciate the most difficult times of your life. How have they made you a better person? How can you use the strong emotions associated with those hard times to promote even more positive change? The strength to radically reinvent yourself is available whenever you embrace it. As soon as you recognize you are free to change, you are charged with the responsibility of doing so. You get exactly one shot at living a human life, and it is a time-limited opportunity. You can alchemize every domain of your life and create your best possible self any time you commit to it. Weigh anchor and get underway!

DAY 3: DON'T PURSUE HAPPINESS

"It is not in the pursuit of happiness that we find fulfillment. It is in the happiness of pursuit."[xix]
~ Seneca

Aging heroes know where we are going because we set a course. Our journey is life itself, and our direction is whichever is most meaningful. For sailors, an up-to-date nautical map is an essential tool for planning a passage. A well-considered personal philosophy is the necessary instrument for aging heroes marking life's course. Creating your philosophy will require a clear mind and an open heart. You should evaluate your ideas from several perspectives to ensure they are sound and represent your highest ideals. One error people sometimes make in determining their philosophies is accepting shallow notions that don't hold up to scrutiny. Using time-worn but poorly thought-out concepts is like relying on an inaccurate, outdated map to plot a course.

You may have heard the story of the little boy who asked his mother why she always cut off the end of the roast before cooking it. The mother answered, "That is just the proper way to prepare a roast. It is how my mother did it." The boy then went to his grandmother and asked why she always cut the end off the roast before cooking it. The grandmother replied, "Because I only had one pot, and it was too small for a full-sized roast." The point is that human beings are prone to automatically assuming the processes and ideas they have been using their whole lives are accurate and effective. A little questioning can reveal some unexpected truths.

Sayings you have heard a million times are sometimes complete bullshit. Think about this old trope: "Book smarts, but no common sense." This saying implies that people who educate themselves tend to have poor judgment in practical matters. While you may have met an egghead or two who couldn't tie his shoes, these exceptions are insignificant. Consider how many book-smart people you know who manage their lives well and demonstrate plenty of common sense. Research shows that intelligence tends to generalize. That means someone smart in one area is likely to be competent in most other areas as well. People with book smarts have *more* common sense than people without them. They typically make better business, relationship, and health decisions.[xx][xxi][xxii] Isn't it common sense to get some book smarts!? "Book smarts, but no common sense" is a sour grapes way for people who feel bad about themselves to take intelligent people down a peg.

Another famous adage that doesn't hold up is, "Those who can, do. Those who can't, teach." This one implies that if an individual is competent, she will employ her skills to make money, and if she is incompetent, she will take a job teaching others those skills. When you hear something enough, it sounds true. But, when you look at this idea more closely, it falls apart. Teaching requires specific talents, just like any other job. Good teachers are knowledgeable in their topic areas, strong communicators, and good motivators. They are organized and thorough, and they are effective classroom managers. A highly skilled lawyer, electrician, or musician could be terrible at teaching those skills to others. Anyone who has ever been a student knows good teachers are relatively rare and have abilities far beyond merely plying the trades they teach.

The nonsense idea that often trips people up when looking for direction in life is summed up in Bobby McFerrin's song, "Don't worry. Be happy." It sounds like a nice sentiment initially, but it doesn't wash. I used to work as a child and family therapist for a community mental health center. When I asked parents what they wanted most for their children, the response was almost universal,

"We just want them to be *happy*." Really? Have you shown them how? Have you mastered the elusive *happy life*? If you haven't been able to pull it off, how on earth can you expect your children to do it? What does it even mean? Has anyone in history ever achieved it? Would anyone even want to? Happiness is an emotion, and emotions are like the weather. They are constantly changing. When you reflect on it, narrowing your life to the single emotion of happiness would be creepy and robotic. Think, *Stepford Wives*.

We are meant to partake in the full range of human experiences. Life is naturally happy, sad, surprising, boring, fascinating, depressing, exciting, and every emotional descriptor imaginable. Anything less would be *less* than human. Motion pictures are not all happy. There are comedies, dramas, love stories, horror movies, action-adventure flicks, documentaries, and tragedies. Deep down, we *want* to emote. Old-fashioned carnivals had a roller coaster to thrill us, a house of mirrors to confuse us, a burlesque show to titillate us, and a haunted house to scare us. A carnival with just one attraction would not be much of a carnival. A human life with only one emotion would not be much of a life.

You may ask, "Am I supposed to enjoy grieving, illness, pain, failure, and all of the other miserable experiences I might go through?" The answer is "no." You are not meant to *enjoy* the bad parts, but you will experience difficulties regardless, so it only makes sense to value even the most negative events. These unhappy times can bring the gifts of maturity, perseverance, wisdom, and empathy. Suffering can help to cultivate the better parts of your nature. A spoiled child who has been granted her every wish is generally unpleasant company. Adults who have been handed everything on a silver platter don't usually have much compassion for others. Hard times temper and transform our characters in the same way that heat tempers and transforms iron into steel. The Roman philosopher Seneca said, "A gem cannot be polished without friction, nor a (person) without trials."[xxiii]

The pursuit of happiness is a fool's errand. While moments of happiness will emerge as side-effects of adventure, creative works, and altruism, pursuing happiness is like chasing the end of a rainbow. Happiness is a poorly considered goal. When determining your direction, shoot for something with a little more substance.

NOTEBOOK ACTIVITY: THINK IT THROUGH

We have all been misguided by weak assumptions. In your notebook, try to come up with some ideas you grew up with that you always took for granted as being true, but didn't hold up when you examined them more closely. Create a habit of scrutinizing long-standing beliefs and making yourself open to changing positions when needed. This is a tall order. Pulling it off will require great flexibility, self-awareness, and maturity.

DAY 4: LAY YOUR COURSE

"Efforts and courage are not enough without purpose and
direction."
~ John F. Kennedy

To lay your course, you must create your philosophy of life. Aim
high and consider your loftiest ideals. Your philosophy will serve as
a compass to guide you through the gales of life.

Every personal philosophy answers three basic questions:
1. What is life all about?
2. How do we screw it up?
3. How can we fix it?

Modern culture provides a cookie-cutter philosophy that most
of us adopt without awareness. According to society, the answers to
the three basic questions are as follows:
1. Life is about finding happiness through commerce.
2. We screw it up by not working, earning, or spending enough.
3. We can fix it by working harder, earning more, and spending
   more.

Accepting society's answers to these questions can be
catastrophic. Following standards set by someone outside of
yourself is the easy route. It is also a choice that will forever make
you a pawn in someone else's game. Again, living other people's
ideals is the top regret of people on their deathbeds. Despite the
risks, most people accept society's ideology because they either don't
realize that there are alternatives or they assume it is accurate
because it is so familiar.

According to our culture, the reasons we are here are to *earn* and to *consume*. These purposes are deeply rooted in us. Erica and I know this is an unhealthy way to define ourselves. But, having the intellectual understanding that our lives are about more than making and spending money did little to change the feeling that buying things would ultimately bring us fulfillment.

After the terrorist attacks of 9/11/2001, the President of the United States advised Americans to conduct business and go shopping. He didn't mention strengthening social bonds, creating positive goals, or doing good in the world, all proven to increase people's sense of well-being.[xxiv] [xxv] [xxvi] I don't think there was any ill intent in the president's instructions after the tragedy. He was just reiterating the message that rains down on us all day, every day, "Buying things will make you happy."

Avarice, the ever-present need for more, is the driving principle behind our culture's philosophy. To put it bluntly, the meaning of life that has been drilled into us is based on greed and selfishness. The meaning and purpose we are programmed to accept leave us in a constant state of covetous hunger. The character, Golem, from *The Lord of the Rings*, who spent his time yearning and plotting to acquire the precious ring, exemplifies the inner world of everyone who blindly accepts society's philosophy. Defining ourselves as earners and consumers is crude and base. We are so much more. We are adventurers on an odyssey to explore the miracle of being alive!

The philosophy society provides is narrow, hollow, and undesirable. It keeps us caged and running on a treadmill. We can do better. Enjoy the following ideas, but do not accept them. Aging heroes think for themselves. Come up with answers that resonate with you. These examples show how a few different thinkers answered the three questions:

Dame Jean Iris Murdoch saw life as an opportunity to move from ignorance to knowledge, from illusion to reality.[xxvii] Human beings' views are impaired by quick judgments based on incomplete information. She uses the example of a mother-in-law whose personal bias automatically causes her to judge her daughter-in-law negatively. By taking the opportunity to get to know the daughter-in-law and by deliberately re-interpreting the daughter-in-law's behavior through a lens of positivity, the mother-in-law moves from the darkness of ignorance to the light of knowledge.

Murdoch answers the three questions as follows:

1. Life is about moving from illusion to reality.
2. We screw up by accepting our snap judgments without examining our motives and without clearly understanding the person or situation we are judging.
3. We fix it through self-examination, taking time to gather information, and being flexible in our attitudes.

Carl Rogers considered that, at our core, human beings are good, and we naturally want to improve ourselves. He said that people are like acorns. In an environment with plenty of sunshine, water, and good soil, a healthy acorn cannot help but become an oak tree. Likewise, in an atmosphere of genuineness (authenticity), empathy, and respect, a healthy human cannot help but become self-actualized. A self-actualized person has become her best possible self by developing her talents and gifts.

Rogers answers the three questions like this:

1. Life is about self-actualization, being all that we can be.
2. We screw up by exposing ourselves to psychologically toxic environments marked by phoniness, selfishness, and disrespect.
3. We fix it by enriching our environments with authenticity, caring, and deference.

Erica and I think that life is exactly what it is supposed to be. We cannot change life, but we can change ourselves. We believe people are tasked with creating purpose and meaning through personal development, service, and gratitude. Because we only get so many trips around the sun, it makes sense to use some time to develop the *self* fully. The *self* is the instrument through which we experience life. Every aspect of the *self* requires development. This means spending time working on mental, spiritual, social, and physical growth. Being of use is fundamental to a deep sense of purpose. Making the world a better place is good for you and everyone in your life. Cultivating gratefulness can help you enjoy a richer existence, stronger relationships, a greater sense of purpose, and improved emotional health. Marcus Aurelius said, "When you arise in the morning, think of what a privilege it is to be alive, to breathe, to think, to enjoy, to love."[xxviii] Gratitude seems an appropriate response to the incredible gift of being alive.

Our answers to the three questions are:

1. Life is exactly what it is supposed to be. Life is always perfectly what it is.
2. We screw it up by thinking life should be other than it is. For example, "My life should be happy (or exciting, or wealthy, or painless, or trouble-free, or wonderful, etc.)."
3. We fix it by viewing life through a lens of profound appreciation and acceptance, by developing ourselves, and by helping others. Every event, positive or negative, is an opportunity to learn, grow, and feel. Gratitude is the polar opposite of selfishness and replaces avarice with satisfaction and generosity.

NOTEBOOK ACTIVITY: CREATE YOUR PERSONAL PHILOSOPHY

Your life's meaning is what makes YOU feel alive and authentic. How do you answer the three questions? Commit some time to this task. Write it down. Hang it on the fridge and read it every day.

Nothing is carved in stone. You can change and modify your answers as you live and learn. Life is a blank canvas. Paint a masterpiece of meaning unique to you, and make it your guiding principle!

What is life all about?

How do we screw it up?

How can we fix it?

DAY 5: LIVE COURAGEOUSLY

"It takes courage to grow up and become who you really are."[xxix]
~ E.E. Cummings

I took a group counseling class in graduate school at The Citadel in Charleston, South Carolina. During each class meeting, we would spend the first hour listening to a lecture and the second hour sitting in a circle as an actual therapy group. I was pretty unsure of myself when I was young and felt intimidated during the group sessions. I don't think I was the only one who felt that way. Each of us wanted to give the impression of being a therapy genius. The resulting group discussions were incredibly stilted. Late in a session, a quiet girl who was probably the youngest student in the class made a comment that highlighted what was happening.

"You people act like you are full of shit," she said in a matter-of-fact tone.

The class went dead silent, then burst into laughter. We all recognized how phony we were being. It was an "emperor has no clothes" moment. After that, participants started being more authentic in group sessions, and the incident became one of my most powerful grad school memories. I admired that girl's courage. She risked rejection by the group to speak the truth, something I would have never done at that time in my life. I made it a personal goal to emulate her behavior from then on (but maybe with a little more tact). Speaking the truth can be a heroic act.

Courage is a trait that has been honored for thousands of years across all cultures. Courageous behavior has several components. First, courage is intentional, not accidental or random. Living with courage is a conscious choice. It is a choice made with a complete understanding of the possible consequences. Second, courage involves personal risk. That risk may be emotional harm, social harm, or physical harm. No courage is required when no risk is involved. Third, courage is motivated by goodness and nobility. Doing the right thing for the wrong reason is not courage. Courage is born of virtue.

The first thing that comes to mind when asked for examples of courage may be the heroism demonstrated by soldiers who risk their lives in combat. Warriors with good hearts, fighting fairly for a noble cause, are indeed courageous. However, sometimes greater courage is required to refrain from fighting. Sitting Bull said, "For us, warriors are not what you think of as warriors... The warrior, for us, is one who sacrifices himself for the good of others. His task is to take care of the elderly, the defenseless, those who cannot provide for themselves, and above all, the children, the future of humanity."[xxx]

I heard a Zen tale about a warlord in feudal Japan who was scouring the countryside, ransacking town after town. One particular village heard of the approaching army, and the residents fled. Everyone left except an elderly Zen master. The Zen master was meditating when the warlord burst into the room with his sword drawn.

The warlord, shocked at the Zen master's calm response to the invasion, questioned the old man, "Don't you realize that the man before you could run you through without blinking an eye?!"

The Zen master replied, "Don't you realize that the man before you could be run through without blinking an eye?"

When I first read this story, I thought the Zen master had risked his life for no purpose. Yet, here I am, nearly two thousand years later, telling his tale of courage. No courage was required of the warlord. Killing an unarmed man is not an act of bravery. Unfathomable courage was required of the old master to face death without blinking. Some of the most courageous people in history stood by their principles in the face of violence. Martin Luther King, Mahatma Gandhi, and Nelson Mandela, to name a few. In your life, it is unlikely that you will be dealing with an angry warlord, but you will find yourself in situations where you have the opportunity to demonstrate courage by taking risks and doing good in the world.

Acting with courage increases your self-confidence. Courageous acts are not committed by the fearless. They are executed by people who act despite their fears. Overcoming your fears empowers you and models self-empowerment for others. Any time you operate outside of your comfort zone, you are showing courage. With courage comes freedom. Fear is limiting. It hems you in. The world becomes spacious and open for the brave. Anais Nin said, "Life shrinks or expands in proportion to one's courage."[xxxi]

NOTEBOOK ACTIVITY: ACTS OF COURAGE

In your notebook, write down times in your life when you were courageous. You may have stuck up for someone who was being bullied or just spoken the truth when it was uncomfortable. How did it feel to act with courage? Also, record times when you had the opportunity to be courageous but failed to do so. How did those experiences feel?

Do one thing that is outside of your comfort zone today. It may be as simple as striking up a conversation with a stranger. Jot down the experience in your notebook. The more often you operate outside your comfort zone, the more spacious and open your life will feel.

DAY 6: STICK TO THE PLAN

"Plan for what is difficult while it is easy; do what is great while it is small."[xxxii]

~ Sun Tzu

Confucious said, "The man who chases two rabbits catches neither."[xxxiii] Erica and I have been guilty of chasing two rabbits regarding health and fitness. We chased the rabbit of a healthy lifestyle and the rabbit of short-term gratification. We have both had periods in our lives when we were extremely fit. She has run marathons, and I have been able to get pretty ripped from lifting weights. However, we also had times when we could not get into the rhythm of the healthy lifestyle we both desired. Laziness, self-indulgence, and other pursuits got in the way. We had a ridiculous number of false starts. We began with good intentions but inevitably lost the thread and returned to unhealthy habits. Sometimes the whole process happened within the same day!

While having choices is a critical component of satisfaction, there is a point where increased choices lead to decreased happiness.[xxxiv] When I worked as a therapist, many of my clients were adolescent boys with ADHD who were getting into trouble at school and sometimes with the law. When individual therapy and parent training was ineffective, I would switch to group therapy. All people are socially influenced. This is especially true of adolescents. When one person gives you an insight about yourself, it is pretty easy to blow off. When an entire group of people gives you that same insight, it is much more difficult to ignore. If individual therapy, parent training, and group therapy all failed, and the kid was at high risk of landing in jail, my treatment of last resort was military school!

A primary issue with people who have ADHD is an inability to navigate distractions. The average person can set a goal and be distracted by other life issues but still eventually reach the goal. When distractions sideline a person with ADHD, he often loses his way and never reaches his goal. Distractions that prevent goal achievement often come from having too many choices. Do I go to class or cut school and go out with my friends? Do I sleep another hour or get up and start the day? Do I study for my test, or do I play video games? Do I party and escape my bad feelings or stay sober and get my work done? When such choices arise, short-term gratification tends to win the day, and responsibilities go to the back burner.

Military school removes choices. Students in a military school don't have the opportunity to choose what clothes they will wear, when they will get up, when they will eat, when they will study, or when they will go to bed. They are held accountable for following a regimen. I never had an ADHD client who did not excel in military school! People with ADHD, and nearly everyone else, respond to external structure.

Ulysses S. Grant was a failed farmer. He was too impatient to wait for crops to grow. He also failed at business. He was too disorganized. However, when he joined the army, he was phenomenally successful. Amid the structure of military life, he rose to the rank of top General and led the Union to victory over the Confederates. After the war, he was elected President of the United States. He went down as one of the worst presidents in history. Not enough structure!

Every day, each of us makes hundreds of tiny decisions that ultimately shape our futures. We choose our food, our drink, our conversations, our media exposure, our activities, and our attitudes. Without external structure, many of us choose short-term gratification and sacrifice long-term success. Historically, my poor choices (which are myriad) were rationalized with, "I'll do better tomorrow."

When Erica and I were stuck in that unhealthy loop, our good intentions just didn't keep us on course. During times of stress, fatigue, and low mood, we defaulted to poor decisions. Trusting our intuitions of the moment inevitably led to bad choices. After many failures, it was clear that we could not trust ourselves to make those tiny decisions. We needed something outside of ourselves. We needed external structure. We needed a PLAN. And we needed to stick to it! A friend of mine shared the strategy of sticking to the plan with me. It worked well for him, so Erica and I decided to try it. After all, we are way too old for military school!

THE PLAN:

Making a plan was probably our biggest stumbling block. While Erica and I processed the plan idea together, we created plans separately to meet our individual needs. I have learned that I am an "all or nothing" kind of guy. My plan reflects this. Erica is a more moderate person by nature, so she made her plan less comprehensive but more flexible. She revises her plan regularly. Think of your plan as your SOP, your standard operating procedure. *Make it your go-to for daily decision-making.*

Here is my plan:

1. Eat healthy food – I know the difference between healthy and unhealthy food and drink. Choose the healthy options, period. It ain't rocket science.
2. Keep healthy hours – A sleepy, overtired me makes terrible choices.
3. Meditate – Every day, no designated amount of time.
4. Exercise – Every day. Do something, anything.
5. Be kind to myself – Always be at least as kind and patient with myself as I am with others.
6. Manage my stress – Make decisions that result in less stress. Choose carefully which media sources I ingest, conversations I participate in, and people I surround myself with. Remind myself that my thoughts and perceptions are 100% responsible for my stress.
7. Develop my mind - Study a foreign language, read

something (fiction or nonfiction), take a class, watch a documentary, or work on a puzzle.

8. Be appreciative – It is impossible to feel gratitude and anger simultaneously. I have many things to be thankful for.
9. Be productive - Every day. Getting things done contributes to a meaningful life.
10. Be creative – Every day. Creative projects make life richer.
11. Communicate love – I get one life. Let the people I love know how I feel every chance I get.
12. Have fun – Every day, at every opportunity. It is possible to have fun with every aspect of PLAN.

Here is Erica's plan:

1. Don't buy candy - Especially not during work hours. Goal: To break the current pattern.
2. Internal harmony - Reduce known stressors (e.g., start the week off with a tidy house) to decrease anxiety and encourage an overall sense of well-being during her busy week.
3. Do something- Whatever is currently relevant. Maybe it is weight loss, physical activity, romance, or addressing health issues. When Erica feels indecisive, she thinks, "Do something." This helps her to focus on and take action on one of these issues.

THOUGHTS THAT CAN
SCREW UP GOOD INTENTIONS

"I'll feel better if I have a drink (or smoke pot or eat some junk food)."

"I'm too tired to do anything."

"I think I'm catching a cold."

"Should I play on Facebook or learn Spanish on Duolingo? Facebook it is!"

"I can't handle these work/relationship/health/financial (pick one) stressors!"

"I'll do it when I am better off financially."

"I feel a little achy. I should skip exercising today."

"Meditation is boring! I don't have time. I'm not getting anything out of it."

As these and other damaging thoughts arise, program yourself to the automatic response, "What does the plan say?" *Make sure your plan has the correct answers!* Develop your plan when you are rational, well-rested, and clear-headed. Think of your typical poor decisions and create a plan that will default you in the right direction. Treat the plan as if it were a military routine. In the military, many life choices are made for you.

When I allow myself to deliberate between a healthy and unhealthy choice, such as, "Do I order a salad or a hamburger?" or "Do I go to the gym or take a break?" I invariably talk myself into the easy but unhealthy choice. That is where I screw up every time. Asking myself, "What does the plan say?" leads me to eat healthily and exercise. Switching off that internal debate by defaulting to "the plan" helps keep Erica and me on the straight and narrow. Another quick trick I use to improve my daily decisions is to ask myself how the *tomorrow me* will judge the choices of the *today me*.

NOTEBOOK ACTIVITY: MAKE YOUR PLAN

You know where you tend to fall off the wagon from living your best life. Please don't use our plans. Take a few minutes, create your own, and record it in your notebook. Know your plan (I repeat mine like a chant during meditation). Memorize it. Own it. Then, all you have to do is STICK TO THE PLAN.

BEING AN EMOTIONAL HERO

"No matter the situation, never let your emotions
overpower your intelligence."
~ Unknown

Emotions evolved because they helped our ancestors survive. Feelings of love and affection motivated ancient people to band together and protect younger and weaker members of their tribes. Anger and fear, associated with the fight or flight response, gave our ancestors the instinct to protect themselves by confronting danger or fleeing to safety. In modern times, some of these primitive instincts can cause problems. Every animal, including humans, has the instinct to trust its gut feelings. For animals in nature, trusting gut feelings is an effective way to survive. However, for a person living in modern society, the instinct to always trust gut feelings and act on emotions can cause trouble.

DAY 7: REFIT YOUR MIND

"Change your thoughts, change your life."[xxxv]
~ Jeanette Coron

I waste a ridiculous amount of time shopping online for used sailboats that I don't intend to buy. The value of a sailboat drops dramatically as it ages. Old boats become less and less functional. The only way for an old sailboat to maintain some of its original value is for the owner to refit, or recondition it. Doing the work to keep a boat up to date takes much time and effort (not to mention money). But new paint, engine, rigging, electronics, and sails can make an old boat pretty attractive to prospective buyers.

Minds that operate with unhealthy or obsolete thought patterns are like sailboats that have fallen into disrepair. Ideas and behaviors that served you well in childhood may be utterly dysfunctional in adult life. For instance, some children got more attention from their parents when they were sick. As adults, a dysfunctional pattern of hypochondriasis may remain. Children who got what they wanted by having tantrums may continue to blow up at people as adults. Without conscious effort, destructive habits can become fixed and predictable, but they do not have to. Folks who allow harmful ideas and behavior patterns to become ingrained are indeed prisoners in cages of their own making. Fortunately, there is a proven strategy for refitting your mind.

There is a Chinese parable about an old farmer whose plow horse ran away. His neighbors sympathetically said, "What bad luck!" The farmer responded, "Maybe."

The next morning the farmer's horse returned accompanied by a herd of wild horses. Now the farmer's stable was full. His neighbors exclaimed, "How lucky you are!" The farmer answered, "Maybe."

The following day the farmer's son fractured his leg trying to break one of the untamed horses. The farmers' neighbors all said, "What terrible luck for this to happen." The farmer said, "Maybe."

The next day war broke out, and all of the fit young men were drafted. The farmer's son was exempt because of his leg injury. The neighbors all congratulated the farmer, "That was good luck!" The farmer once again answered, "Maybe."

Have you ever had an experience that you initially labeled unfavorable but later recognized as very positive? Maybe you had a romantic breakup that seemed like the end of the world, but later, you felt lucky to be free from it. After some time, you realized that the relationship had been toxic. If you have had this or a similar experience, what changed? The event didn't change. *Only your thoughts about that event changed.*

Changing your feelings by changing your thoughts is the underlying principle behind cognitive-behavioral therapy. Cognitive-behavioral therapy, or CBT, is currently the gold standard of counseling therapies. While many therapeutic strategies can be effective, none have as much supporting research as CBT.[xxxvi] Cognitive-behavioral therapy can "alter brain function in patients suffering from major depressive disorder (MDD), obsessive-compulsive disorder, panic disorder, social anxiety disorder, specific phobias, posttraumatic stress disorder, and borderline personality disorder (BPD)."[xxxvii]

The events in your life are neutral and do not affect your emotions. This is hard to wrap your mind around, but it is the objective truth. An event I consider exciting, you might find terrifying. An occurrence that seems emotionally devastating today may wind up feeling completely unimportant when a little time has passed. The positive and negative labels we place on events are *purely subjective.* That is, they are based on opinions and not on facts.

When I first got to know Erica, I assumed she had been through extensive therapy. She had not. When she described her thought processes during stressful events, they were straight from the CBT handbook. Somehow, Erica came to use cognitive behavior therapy techniques with zero knowledge or training! She naturally utilizes her thoughts to reframe situations in ways that improve her life. I suspect that many people of color in the US have developed internal coping mechanisms to deal with the frequent stressors placed on them in our culture. There was an experiment where white Americans were treated in the same stereotypic way that black Americans are treated every day.[xxxviii] Most of the white folks broke down and could not manage the unfair treatment for even a few hours. Erica's go-to in upsetting circumstances is to choose a direction other than upset. She is more concerned with finding a resolution than "winning" in a conflict. She is a kung fu master of defusing emotionally volatile situations.

Erica is a natural when it comes to cognitive behavioral therapy. I am not. I had to learn the techniques and learn to practice them. They are simple to learn, but it takes commitment, creativity, and maturity to put them to use consistently. Cognitive-behavioral therapy is a practical approach to improving emotional health. So, how do you do it?

STEP ONE: IDENTIFY NEGATIVE FEELINGS AND BEHAVIORS

At the top of the next page is a table describing typical reactions to a common frustration, being stuck in traffic. Often our feelings lead us around by the nose, and we emote with little awareness of the process.

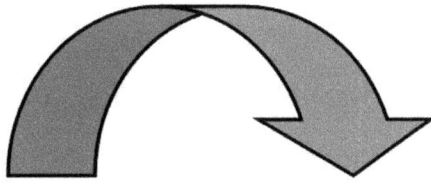

EVENT	FEELINGS AND BEHAVIORS
You are running late and you are stuck in traffic behind a guy who is driving very slow-ly. There is no way to get around him.	Anger
	Frustration
	Anxiety
	Self-Loathing
	Defeated
	Upset Stomach
	Headache
	Heart Palpitations
	Muscle Tension
	Sweating
	Cursing
	Tailgating

The first step in CBT is to **be consciously aware when you are beginning to experience negative emotions.** Name those emotions and notice the behaviors and physical sensations relating to them. Note that the feelings and behaviors create a state of misery.

STEP TWO: IDENTIFY KNEE-JERK IRRATIONAL THOUGHTS

Cognitive-behavioral therapy informs us that *events have absolutely nothing to do with feelings and behaviors,* and if you were the person experiencing being late and stuck in traffic per the table below, the actual cause of your wretched responses would be *your thoughts.* This is important because, while you have no control over external events, you are capable of changing your thoughts about those events.

NEUTRAL

EVENT	THOUGHTS AND PERCEPTIONS	FEELINGS AND BEHAVIORS
You are running late and you are stuck in traffic behind a guy who is driving very slowly. There is no way to get around him.	I'm going to get in trouble! I always do this! That guy can't drive! He's an idiot! He's a jerk! I can't take it any more This is terrible!	Anger Frustration Anxiety Self-Loathing Defeated Upset Stomach Headache Heart Palpitations Muscle Tension Sweating Cursing Tailgating

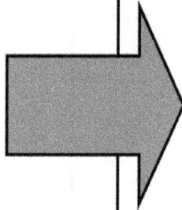

*The second step in CBT is to **recognize the irrational thoughts and perceptions that are causing your emotional responses**.* Write them down. Some underlying assumptions that are almost always present when negative emotions emerge are, "I can't take it anymore," and "This is terrible!"

STEP THREE: FORCEFULLY CHALLENGE IRRATIONAL THOUGHTS

The core process in CBT is to vigorously challenge irrational thoughts that arise in stressful situations. Your ego will be the most significant barrier to success because your thoughts naturally *feel* true, and you are wired to believe what feels true. *A primary human thinking error is to mistake feeling true for being true.*

NEUTRAL

EVENT	THOUGHTS AND PERCEPTIONS	CHALLENGES
You are running late and you are stuck in traffic behind a guy who is driving very slowly. There is no way to get around him.	I'm going to get in trouble! →	Unless it is a chronic problem, people rarely get in trouble for being late.
	I always do this! →	No you don't.
	That guy can't drive! →	You can't possibly know that from one observation.
	He's an idiot! →	He may be a genius.
	He's an asshole! →	He may be driving to the hospital to donate a kidney.
	I can't take it any more →	Oh yeah? What else are you going to do? You have "taken" much worse than this in your life
	This is terrible! →	Cancer is terrible. Being late is inconvenient.

In step three, you **create logical challenges to each irrational thought**. This is the most difficult part of the cognitive behavior therapy process because it is human nature to trust our thoughts regardless of how ludicrous they may be. One strategy that may help is to pretend they are someone else's irrational thoughts and you are helping them come up with challenges. Write down the cognitive challenges and remember that these rational interpretations are true regardless of whether or not they feel true. *CBT* **will not work if you fail to successfully complete step three.**

Q: "What if my thoughts ARE true? What if I know the guy in the car, and he IS a stupid asshole?"

A: Do you want to continue to be miserable? Failing to forcefully challenge your thoughts will keep you trapped in a hell of your own making. If you know the guy is a stupid asshole, question the logic of your reactions to that truth. As you stew in your toxic emotions, the idiot jerk is enjoying a nice slow drive to where ever he is going.

In a situation over which you have no control, is it rational for you to make yourself miserable? Is it logical to carry on like a three-year-old? Besides, haven't you been the slow, preoccupied driver at some point in your past? The only rational response to this situation over which you have no control is to take a deep breath, turn on your favorite music, and enjoy the ride.

Note the human tendency to judge our behaviors in a different way than we judge other people's behaviors. When we behave badly, we do so for a good reason. When others misbehave, we assume it is because they are bad people. When I cut someone off in traffic, it is not because I am bad. It is because my situation warranted me cutting someone off. But when someone cuts me off in traffic, it's because that person is a jerk. Marcus Aurelius said, "When faced with people's bad behavior, turn around and ask when you have acted like that."

STEP FOUR: FEEL PROUD OF YOUR CHANGED FEELINGS AND BEHAVIOR

NEUTRAL

EVENT	THOUGHTS AND PERCEPTIONS	CHALLENGES	FEELINGS AND BEHAVIORS
You are running late and you are stuck in traffic behind a guy who is driving very slowly. There is no way to get around him.	I'm going to [obscured] I a[obscured] this! [obscured] guy ca[obscured]! an idiot! [obscured] asshole! I ca[obscured]t any more This is terrib[obscured]	Unless it is a chronic problem, people rarely get in trouble for being late. No you don't. You can't possibly know that from one observation. He may be a genius. He may be driving to the hospital to donate a kidney. Oh yeah? What else are you going to do? You have "taken" much worse than this in your life Cancer is terrible. Being late is inconvenient.	You feel ok. Turn on your favorite radio station and enjoy the ride like a rational human being!

In step four, be aware of the changes in emotions you created. **Experience the power of your abilities.** Feel proud that you moved from a childish response to a mature one. Imagine a magical world where you have rewired your knee-jerk reactions to unpleasant events. You are 100% capable of making this happen! That first negative ping of irritation should be your cue to start challenging your thoughts. Don't wait until you are in the throes of emotion. Intense emotional states tend to short-circuit the rational mind. In sailing, reefing is when you decrease the size of a sail by drawing it in a little and tying it off. Reefing is done to make sailing in strong winds a little safer. The saying is to "reef early and reef often." In cognitive-behavioral therapy, we say, "challenge your thoughts early and challenge your thoughts often!"

NOTEBOOK ACTIVITY: WORK YOUR CBT

A CBT therapist would give you weekly homework to complete steps one through four on paper using stressful situations from your own life. Use your notebook and try it right now. Commit to working through your negative emotions in writing until the process becomes natural and automatic. *Begin by working through the steps every time negative emotions arise for the rest of this 30-day voyage.* This is a tall order, but it is crucial. Use as many pages as you need and insert them into your notebook whenever the opportunity arises.

The key is to attack toxic thoughts with cognitive challenges and never give in to the natural inclination to buy into those thoughts. If you run into a snag, get a friend to help. Be very specific when you ask your friend for assistance. You want help challenging your thoughts. If your friend agrees with your irrational thoughts, she is not helping. Ask someone else. Sometimes, other people can recognize our irrational thoughts much better than we can. Over time, you can rewire your brain so that your responses will be healthy and adaptive rather than immature and destructive.

- Step One: Identify Negative Feelings and Behaviors
- Step Two: Identify Knee-Jerk Irrational Thoughts
- Step Three: Vigorously Challenge Irrational Thoughts
- Step Four: Feel Proud of Your Changed Feelings and Behaviors

When the cartoon GI Joe says, "Knowing is half the battle,"[xxxix] he is wrong. I first learned about cognitive-behavioral therapy in graduate school and thought at the time that this knowledge would change my life. It didn't. My life did not change until I started practicing CBT over and over every single day. Possessing CBT knowledge is not transformative. *Applying* the knowledge is. You can improve every aspect of your life, from relationships to fitness to emotional health! All you have to do is start practicing. Make a lifelong habit of challenging negative thoughts.

DAY 8: MANAGE BAD DAYS

"Negative emotional states are a breeding ground for mistakes."[xl]
~ Sam Owen

Gut feelings are necessary for us to navigate life. They give us a shortcut for decision-making. Our gut feelings are accurate much of the time. Unfortunately, this gives us the false sense that they are always right. They are not.

Your gut feelings are out of whack when you have a bad day. Because they evolved from survival instincts, gut feelings can easily overwhelm the higher intellect. Strong emotions can override good judgment. When we are amid intense emotional states, we are most likely to say and do things we later regret. Pythagoras said, "In anger, we should refrain from both speech and action."[xli]

Although it is perfectly natural to assume your feelings are accurate, this assumption becomes a HUGE problem when your gut feelings give you bad information. Messages from your gut when you are having an off day can look like this:

"Nobody likes me."

"He is a jerk!"

"I can tell she meant that as an insult."

"I am a failure."

"He is trying to make me angry."

"Everyone can see that I am a loser."

"These things always happen to *me*!"

Your negative mood escalates when you trust the false messages that you are no good or that the people around you are not good. Reeling negative emotions back in at a certain point is next to impossible. Trying to work through a problem when your feelings are out of control is pointless. Thinking your way out of rage or extreme sadness is like thinking your way out of a bad cold. You can be aware that you have a cold and think positive, healthy thoughts, but you will still have a cold. Strong emotions always pass, but they usually do so gradually.

The best way to handle negative emotions is to catch them early before they become so overpowering that you can't control them. Be self-aware. Pay close attention to internal cues that you are getting upset. That is the time to use your CBT techniques from Day 7 or to simply take a time out. One red flag that lets me know I am in a bad mood is when I start blaming my unhappiness on others. I may get agitated at Erica because I can't find my glasses, or I get angry at the universe when my car doesn't start.

When I know I am in a bad state, I inform Erica and then find some distraction. I might watch a movie, go for a walk, take a nap, or head for the lake. Erica and I understand that other priorities must be put on hold if either of us is in a bad mental state. We work very hard to monitor our own emotions and communicate them with each other. The message usually goes something like this, "I love you. This has nothing to do with you. I am in a bad headspace and need to check out for a while." This may be a difficult message to receive if you are the other partner. You might feel unsatisfied because putting the issue on hold is not meeting your immediate needs. On a gut level, you also may not believe that the issue needs to be tabled until later. Get over it! For this strategy to work, both partners must do their part. Erica and I are experienced enough to accept this kind of communication at face value, move on to something else, and not take it personally. When we are both on board with the strategy, it works like a charm and keeps us on an even keel.

Erica and I sat down and discussed why this technique works so well for us and what barriers might keep it from working for others. We believe that one obstacle is an imbalance of power. Erica and I are complete individuals with or without each other. What we have is not built on codependency. Neither of us needs the other to be a whole person. Our relationship is genuinely equal. We don't just give lip service to that idea. The distribution of power between us is even. We still recognize that each of us has different strengths and weaknesses, so we take on responsibilities accordingly. Some of these responsibilities conform to common gender norms, and some don't. But, the undercurrent of our relationship is always about mutual respect. Neither of us needs or desires to be parented by the other. We have both been in relationships where power was unequal. A boat with an uneven distribution of weight is a dangerous vessel. A relationship where power is off-center is an unhealthy one. If one partner considers themself superior to the other, the communication strategy Erica and I use will likely fail.

Having a strategy in your relationship for managing when one partner is in a bad emotional place is essential. Likewise, each of us needs a personal approach to deal with our emotions when they are off-kilter. One thing I do is ease up on myself and other people. I pay attention to my self-talk. Are the things I am saying to myself comforting, or do they make matters worse? As soon as I become aware that I am in a bad space, I consciously start to shift my inner dialogue:

"Take it easy. I can't trust my feelings right now."

"This is not the right time for me to make big decisions or judgments about my life."

"Negative emotions are like thunderstorms. They will eventually move on."

"If these same things happened on a day when I was in a good mood, they would not affect me at all."

"I am in a bad mood, and it is nobody's fault. It is not fair to blame others for how I am feeling."

When I realize I am dealing with strong emotions, my priorities shift. I know the machine I use for problem-solving, planning, and social interactions is malfunctioning, so it's the wrong time to engage in those activities.

NOTEBOOK ACTIVITY: MANAGING YOUR BAD DAYS

Make a plan for how you will manage your next bad day and record it in your notebook. Steal whatever you need from this and previous chapters. Make a mental note to return to your notebook and implement your plan as soon as you recognize that you are having a bad day. Managing emotions requires recognizing emotions. If you are not self-aware, you will be the slave of your feelings rather than the master of them. Managing your emotions well radiates out to the rest of the world. Not only do you make life easier for the people you interact with, but you also model for them what it looks like to be a mature adult.

DAY 9: CHOOSE OPTIMISM

"Optimism is essential to achievement, and it is also the foundation of courage and true progress."[xlii]
~ Nicholas M. Butler

Converting from pessimism to optimism is an absolute necessity if you want to live a long, healthy life. I was a card-carrying pessimist as a young man. Thankfully, I reformed. Optimism is directly related to improved success socially, mentally, physically, and even vocationally.[xliii] Ultimately, optimists enjoy far more achievements in life than pessimists. Optimism lowers your chance of developing heart disease by 35% and decreases your likelihood of early death by 14%.[xliv] Blood sugar, cholesterol, and risks for cancer and infection are all lower in optimists.[xlv xlvi]

Beginning in 1930, a fascinating study was conducted involving Catholic nuns.[xlvii] Before taking their final vows, each of the 180 sisters was asked to write a short essay about her life, including important events and what brought her to join the convent. Seventy years later, researchers used a coding system to classify each essay as either optimistic or pessimistic. Amazingly, the nuns who had written optimistic essays 70 years earlier lived nearly ten years longer than the other sisters in the study!

As a young, depressive pessimist, I could point out incidents from history, current events, and my own life to support my negative outlook. Unfortunately, such evidence is so abundant that the average pessimist will claim to be a *realist* rather than a pessimist. Make no mistake, neither optimists nor pessimists are realists. Reality is *objective*. It exists independent of the mind. If I am standing behind a table that holds two bowls of ice cream and I say, "I have two bowls of ice cream in front of me." That is a statement of *objective* fact. My statement reflects reality. The fact that the bowls of ice cream are in front of me does not depend on my feelings or beliefs to be true. However, if I say chocolate ice cream is better than vanilla, I am making a *subjective* statement. This subjective statement depends on my thoughts and feelings about chocolate and vanilla. Optimism and pessimism are subjective. They rely on opinion, not on external reality.

Have you ever wondered why the news in the media has more negative stories than positive ones? Well, it turns out that human beings gravitate to what is called a *negative bias.*[xlviii] That is, we pay much more attention to negative than positive information. This was once an adaptive trait. It helped early people survive. Adverse events were more likely to be life-threatening for primitive humans thousands of years ago. The cave people who paid attention and learned from adverse events were likelier to stay alive long enough to have children and pass on their genes. We evolved to tune into negative situations. No wonder pessimism abounds!

The good news is that optimism is a conscious choice, a habit. I am living proof that a pessimist can be converted. As a young pessimist, I had a negative view of humanity. As an old optimist, I realize that the number of times people have been kind and supportive in my life dwarfs the number of times people have been unpleasant. Have people been more positive than negative in your life? If not, can you identify the role you might have played in your negative experiences? Do negative situations seem to happen more in your life than in other people's lives?

There was a fun experiment I used to do with my classes. I asked them to look around the room and take note of everything that was the color blue. I gave them a minute to look around, and then I would ask everyone to close their eyes and try to recall everything in the room that was yellow. Everyone always laughed at how difficult it was to remember yellow items. The lesson was that we find what we look for. Look for the positive in the world, and you will find the world is positive. Look for the negative in the world, and you will indeed find that the world is negative.

A North American folk tale tells of a traveler who happened upon an old woman washing clothes in a stream. The traveler stopped and asked her, "What are the people in the next town like?"

The old woman looked up from her work and said, "Well, what were the people like in your town?"

The traveler responded, "They were just awful. Every one of them was a lying, selfish jackass."

"Oh, I am afraid you will find the same is true in the next town," said the old woman shaking her head. The disappointed traveler went on his way, mumbling under his breath.

A few minutes later, another traveler approached the old woman and asked the same question, "What are the people like in the next town?"

Again, the old woman replied with the question, "What were the people like in your town?"

"They were wonderful. Some of the finest people you could ever hope to meet" answered the second traveler.

The old woman grinned, "I am pleased to say that you will find the same kind of people in the next town."

The wise old woman demonstrated an innate understanding of what J.W. Goethe was communicating when he said, "A man sees in the world what he carries in his heart."[xlix]

If you, like me, find the people in your life to be more positive than negative, can you generalize that perception to people everywhere? Humans naturally tend to divide others into two groups, *us* (people like me) and *them* (people not like me). We tend to judge people we consider "us" favorably and people we view as "them" unfavorably. However, research disputes assumptions drawn from the "us and them" mentality. It shows that human beings are pretty much the same the world over. We all want better lives for ourselves, our friends, and our families. All of us want to be loved and appreciated, and we want to be safe and successful.

Choosing optimism may be easier than you think. Data from across the globe shows the same patterns. Life satisfaction decreases from childhood until around mid-life, then steadily increases from mid-life to death.

AGE AND LIFE SATISFACTION

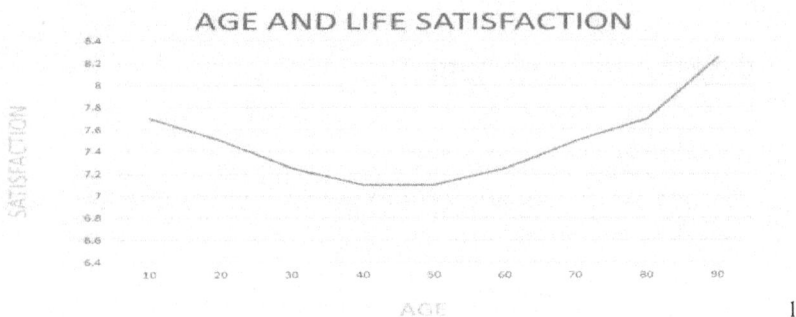

The reverse pattern happens with stress. Stress rises from childhood to middle age and decreases from middle age to death.

NOTEBOOK ACTIVITY: USE COGNITIVE-BEHAVIORAL THERAPY TO CHOOSE OPTIMISM

Use your four CBT steps to attack your pessimistic beliefs. Choosing optimism is a habit that requires practice and self-awareness. To flip your cynical worldview, you must repeatedly challenge your thoughts until optimism becomes your natural go-to. The only obstacle to making the change from pessimism to optimism is your ego.

Part 1: Ask yourself the following questions, then challenge any pessimistic answers using the four steps of cognitive-behavioral therapy:

- Do you expect good things to happen in your future, or are you waiting for the other shoe to drop? Why?

- Do you think other people are good or bad? Why?
- Do you think others view you in a positive light or a negative one? Why?

Part 2: If any of your answers were pessimistic, use the four CBT steps from Day 7 to challenge them:
- Step One: Identify the negative feelings relating to your pessimistic answers
- Step Two: Restate the negative thoughts in your pessimistic answers
- Step Three: Vigorously challenge those thoughts as irrational and unproductive
- Step Four: Feel Proud of the changed feelings and behaviors that resulted from dispelling those unhealthy ideas

Marianne Williamson said, "personal transformation can and does have global effects. As we go, so goes the world, for the world is us. The revolution that will save the world is ultimately a personal one."[li] Override your ego and improve your life and the lives of everyone who comes in contact with you.

DAY 10: CONVERT YOUR STRESS

"A crust eaten in peace is better than a banquet partaken in anxiety."
~ Aesop

The human stress reaction comes from the *fight-or-flight response*, a hardwired survival trait that has kept us in the gene pool for thousands of years. Life was uncertain for primitive people living in nature. They had to deal with wild animals trying to eat them and aggressive neighbors trying to wipe them out. Those who responded to threats with violence (fight) or by running away (flight) survived to raise offspring. They passed on their genes. All animals have a fight-or-flight response. If a child tries to catch a squirrel, the squirrel will run away (flight). If by some miracle, the child could grab the squirrel before it ran away, it would undoubtedly bite the child (fight).

Erica and I took a wonderful trip to Africa a few years ago and went on a safari at the Ngorongoro Crater. The experience was surreal. It was extraordinary to see exotic animals living freely in their natural habitats. There were lions, flamingos, zebras, elephants, giraffes, wildebeests, baboons, and hippos. When we arrived, we could see a tribe of Maasai sitting around a campfire in the far distance. The Maasai are transhumance pastoralists, meaning they survive by herding cows and goats from place to place. They are famously courageous. I asked our guide if the Maasai feared lions and other predators. He answered, "The lions are afraid of the Maasai!"

When a predator, like a hungry lion, springs into action against a herd of grazing gazelles, the herd's fight-or-flight response kicks in, and they run away. If the lion is lucky, it may catch one of the weaker members of the herd and have a meal. What do the other gazelles do immediately after the threat has passed? They go back to grazing!

Imagine a similar situation, but instead of a herd of gazelles, it is a football team having practice. The lion again springs into action, chases the team, and eats one of the players. Do you think the surviving team members would go back to having practice? No, they would probably be in therapy for the rest of their lives!

The fight-or-flight response is meant to operate as it does in the gazelle herd, not the football team. It is supposed to turn on when there is a threat and turn off when the danger has passed. Unfortunately, one side effect of having the most highly developed brain on the planet is that we respond to memories of threats and imaginary threats in the same way as we do to actual threats. We invent LOTS of imaginary threats! In modern life, most of us are rarely in situations where our lives are in real danger, so in the absence of lions and poisonous snakes, we stress over things that our ancestors would consider absurd. Our fight-or-flight response is triggered by bills, schoolwork, jobs, and relationship issues. The result for many modern people is a near-constant state of stress!

Like humans, baboon troops have a pecking order. At the top of the pecking order is the strongest, most aggressive baboon, and at the bottom is the weakest and most passive. There is a direct relationship between stress and the relative health of baboons as one moves up and down the pecking order. The baboon at the top enjoys the best food, the first pick of sexual partners, and the most physical attention from others in the troop. The top baboon also has the lowest stress levels and the most robust health. As you move down the pecking order, stress increases, and health decreases. Baboons at the bottom of the pecking order are likely to suffer from high blood pressure, arthritis, diabetes, and obesity.[lii]

The same is true for humans. People at the top of the pecking order in their jobs, likewise, experience less stress, report more joy, and have the best health. People with jobs at the bottom of the pecking order tend to have higher levels of stress and poorer health. Low-end workers take far more sick leave than people working in upper management.[liii] If you are in a job at the lower end of the pecking order, one solution would be to find social outlets that allow you to be on the high end of a pecking order. You might organize a book club, volunteer to chair a committee, or run for president of a local civic club.

While the stress response is beneficial in the natural environment, it can wreak havoc in modern life. Long-term stress can result in cardiovascular disease, obesity, alcoholism, asthma, accelerated aging, diabetes, Alzheimer's disease, digestive disorders, depression, anxiety, pain, and premature death![liv] Understanding the long-term health risks of chronic stress can cause a lot of stress! Here is the caveat. Your mindset affects the way your body responds to stress.[lv] People who experience a lot of pressure but view stress as life-enhancing or positive have fantastic health outcomes. Their health is not only much better than people who have a lot of stress and view it as debilitating, but also better than people who have low stress! This relates to optimism. Optimism overrides even the destructive health effects of chronic stress and transforms high stress into a health enhancer!

So, your number one tool for combating the adverse effects of stress is optimism. What else can you do to manage stress? Here are a few strategies:

- *Exercise.* The fight or flight response prepares the body to fight or run. While fighting when you are stressed will likely land you in jail, running can decrease your stress and improve your cardiovascular fitness. If you don't like to run, any activity that gets your heart pumping will work, even sex!
- *Breathe.* If you take a yoga, martial arts, or meditation class, you will find that they usually start with

breathwork. The fight or flight stress response is part of the autonomic nervous system, which controls your heart rate, blood pressure, breath rate, digestion, and other body functions that take place automatically. Hence, the name autonomic. Most of these functions are beyond your control. If asked to slow your heart rate, you would probably be unable to do that. However, you do have some control over your breath. Breath, heart rate, and blood pressure are all connected, so when you take slow, deep breaths, your heart rate and blood pressure naturally decrease. Take a deep breath, hold it for a few seconds, and then release it in a slow sigh. You should feel more physically relaxed and less anxious immediately.

- *Talk.* Sharing your feelings with a trusted person is highly therapeutic and anxiety-reducing. This effect is called catharsis and is one reason people feel better after a talk therapy session.

- *Write.* Have you ever been lying in bed with your mind reeling about something that upset you? You may have found that you replayed the upsetting event over and over. One easy strategy for letting the obsession go is to write down your thoughts. Writing out whatever you were ruminating over allows the mind to release it. It is almost like saving a document on your computer. Once it is saved, you don't have to worry about it anymore. You don't need to do anything with what you wrote. The act of writing it down is what does the trick.

- *Listen.* Music can be a fantastic tool for decreasing stress. You already know this intuitively. You have listened to slow music that relaxed you, and you have heard fast music that got your blood moving. There is a scientific reason for this. Different mental states produce different brain waves. Long, slow brain waves happen when you are calm and relaxed. Short, fast brain waves are generated when you are alert and excited. Music, likewise, produces waves, soundwaves. Brainwaves tend to synchronize with soundwaves. Long, slow soundwaves synchronize with the brain and create long, slow brain waves.

NOTEBOOK ACTIVITY: MANAGE YOUR STRESS

Choose one or more of the stress management strategies listed above and commit to using them for the next 20 days. Keep track of your success in your notebook. Try new strategies until you find what works for you, then make that strategy a habit.

BEING AN INTELLECTUAL HERO

"Intellectual growth should commence at birth and cease only at death."[lvi]
~ Albert Einstein

Your intellect can be developed just like your physical body. Nearly anyone willing to put in the work can make dramatic improvements to their physical bodies. The same is true for folks willing to work to develop their minds. Without intentional development, the mind can become sluggish, dull, and brittle. Poorly developed minds can lead to behaviors and attitudes that cause harm. Numerous strategies can help you keep your mind nimble, creative, flexible, and open to learning.

DAY 11: DEVELOP INSIGHT

"A point of view can be a dangerous luxury when substituted for insight and understanding"
~ Marshall McLuhan

There is a Chinese story about a robber who stole a great bell from the town square. Because the bell was so big and heavy, the thief had to carry it on his back. Every time he took a step, the bell rang loudly. Afraid that the noise would draw attention and cause him to get caught, the robber tore pieces from his shirt and stuffed them in his ears so he could no longer hear the ringing. "There, that's better," he thought, proud of his cleverness.

What should be evident to anyone reading the story, that everyone else could still hear the bell, was not apparent to the bell thief. The robber lacked insight. The bell thief was misguided. However, like the bell thief, we all have blind spots where we lack insight. These blind spots are apparent to the people in our lives but invisible to us. Worse, we often remain in the dark even when multiple people try to inform us about them!

Early in our relationship, Erica told me I had anger issues. Anger issues!? I told her she was crazy. I am one of the nicest, kindest, most even-tempered guys around. She said, "True, but you also have anger problems." After nearly being arrested for assault when I overreacted to a bully at a movie theater and having several other people confirm Erica's perceptions, I eventually recognized that I indeed had anger problems. Insight is such a weird thing. Developing insight requires taking other people's observations about you seriously. The ego, "I know more about me than anyone," is the greatest obstacle to developing accurate insight. This is especially true in intelligent people who are otherwise good at problem-solving.

I have well-controlled major depression. A combination of excellent medical treatment and a lifetime of accumulated coping strategies have made mood disorder a minor for me. This has not always been the case. For my first 28 years, I felt like a screw-up. I had horrible insomnia, problems with attention and concentration, low energy, tremendous guilt, and frequent thoughts of killing myself. I worked very hard to get control of my life. I tried running, religion, meditation, weightlifting, veganism, all kinds of supplements, talk therapy, self-hypnosis, yoga, and every self-help book I could find. I started each intervention with great hope then I would crash. Depression is tricky because it is cyclic. This made it easy for me to mistakenly think that an intervention was working when I was actually just experiencing the non-depressed part of a mood cycle.

Fortunately, I worked with a medical doctor who insisted on trying me on an antidepressant. I was completely against this and did not believe I had a mental illness. Each of us is trapped in the bubble of our perceptions. The mood disorder warped my perceptions. What I could not see was blatantly apparent to the doctor. I like to compare mental illness to lousy vision. If you have never seen the world through eyes with 20/20 vision, you assume that blurry is how things are supposed to look. When I got my first pair of glasses, I was shocked to find that stars in the night sky were little pinpoints of light and not little fuzzy blobs of light. Before medical treatment, I lacked insight. I assumed that my negative perceptions about life were accurate. I also believed that taking medication somehow spoke to my character, as if accepting medical treatment meant I was weak or incompetent.

At any rate, I complied with the doctor's recommendation and tried the antidepressant. Within a couple of weeks, my mental processes became clear, my sleep and appetite improved dramatically, and my overall functioning skyrocketed. I changed from being the lowest producer in my office to the highest. I returned to grad school and found that instead of struggling for C's,

I easily made A's. This was how "normal" people felt!?! I had been dragging a boulder behind me while everyone else skipped along in life, unaware of how easy they had it!

Now I finally had insight into my condition and enjoyed a normal life, right? Wrong. Antidepressant medications are different from other meds. Their effects are subtle and happen over weeks instead of hours. You do not perceive the obvious cause and effect that you do from aspirin, Xanax, or even beer. Take an aspirin, and your headache will go away. Take Xanax, and you will feel relaxed. Drink a beer, and you will feel slightly tipsy. Being on antidepressants made me *feel* like the circumstances of my life had improved, not that my neurochemistry had improved. As a result, I had to try going off the medicine numerous times before my slow-to-learn ego accepted that I do have a medical condition. Once stable on medication, the other interventions I had tried earlier were able to take root. Diet, exercise, and meditation became terrific tools for improving my life.

High blood pressure can cause heart disease. Imagine a doctor who treated the heart disease but not the high blood pressure. That is basically what I was doing when I tried lifestyle changes without first treating my medical condition.

When I suffered depressive spells, I always turned my negative feelings on myself. "Why am I such a screw-up? Why can't I be like everyone else?" I assumed my misery was because I was a loser. I had an acquaintance who also suffered from depression, but he turned his negative emotions outward. When he had a depressive episode, he assumed his inner suffering was because he lived in a world full of fools. His depression did not make him sad. It made him angry. Imagine how difficult it was for him to accept medical treatment for depression. I called his doctor on the down low and told him I thought his anger was a manifestation of depression. Fortunately, my friend's doctor could talk to him about antidepressants in a way that didn't scare him off. My friend told me years later how much the medication helped him.

I met a lady who had had multiple jobs. Every single one of her bosses over the years was a jerk. Every single business she worked for mistreated her. It never occurred to her that she was the common denominator. What does it look like to be on the other side of you? How might your lack of insight create problems in your life? Do your conflicts have a theme? Do you experience the same relationship issues with lots of different people? Everyone has blind spots. If you believe you are the exception, you are not unique. You are simply one of many who lack insight about your lack of insight!

One strategy to help you develop better insight is to compare your actions to your values. No excuses or rationalizations for your behavior are acceptable. Consider this. Do you believe stealing is wrong? Hopefully, yes. Are you a thief? Hopefully, no. If you put a dollar in a vending machine and it spit out five dollars in change, would you keep it or try to find its rightful owner? Despite a firm belief that stealing is wrong, most of us would keep the five dollars. Now change the situation slightly. The machine gives you five dollars in change, and the owner of the machine is standing next to it. Do you keep the five dollars in this situation? Most of us would not. The difference between our stated value and actual behavior in this situation shows an insight blind spot.

NOTEBOOK ACTIVITY: ASK A FRIEND

Ask someone close to you to help you find your blind spots. Ask them to be kind but brutally honest. Thank them for their help. Write down what you discovered. Also, note ways you may have mentally tried to reject the information your friend or loved one provided. To move forward, you must assume that she gave you honest feedback and then work on whatever issue was uncovered.

DAY 12: AMP UP YOUR INTELLECT

"The brain is like a muscle. When it is in use, we feel very good.
Understanding is joyous."
~ Carl Segan

Erica and I are fanatics about learning. New information and new mental skills help keep our minds agile and fresh. The learning process enables us to adapt to the inevitable changes in our lives as we grow older. It was once believed that if you lived long enough, you would eventually become senile. This is not true. There are certain areas of cognitive decline as you age, but also areas with the potential for continued improvement across the lifespan. Fluid intelligence is the ability to solve unfamiliar problems without a frame of reference. Fluid intelligence begins to decline in young adulthood and continues to decrease as you age. Crystallized intelligence is the ability to use what you have learned. Crystalized intelligence tends to increase as you age. Your vocabulary, for instance, has the potential to become larger and larger.[lvii]

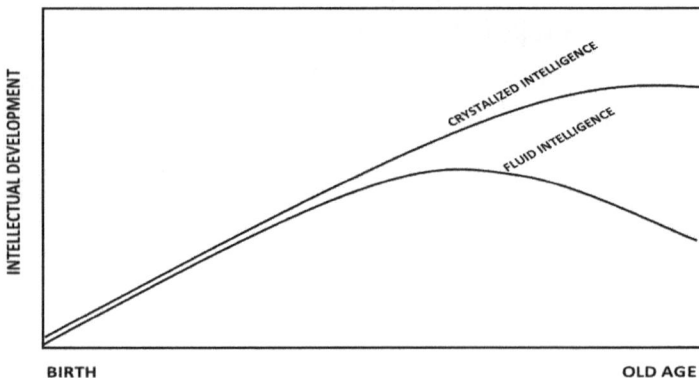

The first step in amping up your intellect is learning and practicing logic. In simple terms, logic is a process for accepting only ideas that can be proven. Proof requires evidence. There is logic to math problems. To prove 1+2=3, put an apple on the table and two more beside it. Now, count all of the apples. If the number you end up with is 3, then you just proved that 1+2=3.

There is logic to the arrangement of the parts that make an engine, an electrical circuit, a computer, and even a simple door latch. The proof of the logic is shown by how well the finished products work. A door latch won't latch properly if the parts are arranged illogically.

Science is applied logic. Look around you right now. If you are not in the middle of a forest, chances are nearly everything you see ultimately resulted from science. The profound impact science has had on human life cannot be overstated. If you stick to an idea that is opposed by science, you likely have an intellectual blind spot, an area of your intellect that probably needs some work.

Second, and equally as important as logic, is objectivity. Why would you stubbornly hold on to an illogical belief or one that is disputed by vast amounts of scientific evidence? The answer is simple, emotions. Emotions evolved to help early humans survive. Trusting our emotional gut feelings is hardwired into us. Without training and practice, your emotions will have a much more significant influence over your choices than your intellect. Because emotions evolved as a survival mechanism, they easily override the intellect. From an evolutionary standpoint, our incredible human intellect was a tremendous upgrade but not much of a survival feature. Scientists are still unsure why we have such advanced brains. We didn't need evolved brains capable of calculus and rocket building. We only required enough brain development to find food and shelter and to protect ourselves.

Emotions are closely related to another human survival trait, egocentrism. Egocentric means that we tend to look out for number one and aren't very good at understanding things from other people's perspectives. Every animal on earth, including humans, tries to protect the *self*. Even a mosquito will fly away when you try to swat it. It is our nature to see the world in terms of the *self* as it relates to everything that is *not the self*. So, when we run into illogical information that makes the *self* feel safe and supported, we tend to accept it as accurate. When logic and evidence conflict with a belief that makes the *self* feel good, it is called *cognitive bias*. Cognitive bias is a massive barrier to intellectual development.

The scientific method is a series of steps designed to factor out cognitive bias and emotional attachments to specific ideas. Compare the volume of human knowledge before and after the scientific revolution. This should make it crystal clear that survival traits that worked so well for so long, namely always trusting our gut feelings and emotions, also kept us from moving forward and accurately understanding our world.

Here are a few proven ways to improve your intellect:

- Play games that require using your memory, problem-solving, or spatial skills. Chess, crosswords, sudoku, and jigsaw puzzles all fit the bill.[lviii] [lix] [lx]
- Meditate. Meditation has been shown to have a positive effect on cognitive processing. Studies have found that meditators tend to have higher IQs than non-meditators.[lxi]
- Learn a new language. All learning creates new neural connections.[lxii]
- Learn a musical instrument. Research has shown a positive relationship between learning music and increasing IQ.[lxiii]
- Exercise. Physical exercise has been found to improve cognitive abilities.[lxiv] The brain is, after all, a bodily organ that benefits when your overall health improves.
- Read. Fiction and non-fiction reading have been shown to improve memory, vocabulary, and even emotional

intelligence.[lxv] Reading books that are a little difficult can have an impact if you take the time to look up terms with which you are unfamiliar.

NOTEBOOK ACTIVITY: GIVE UP ONE EMOTION-BASED BELIEF

In your notebook, identify a belief you have that is rooted in emotion and opposed by evidence that you would be willing to give up. Maybe you think your favorite football team is the greatest of all time, but the statistics point to another team. Perhaps you think your hometown is the best town in America, but your town doesn't measure up when you look at its education levels, employment rates, economic growth, cost of living, and quality of life. A developed intellect requires a willingness to bypass your ego's emotional needs and accept information that may *feel* uncomfortable. This is a tall order, and it requires a lifetime of practice. Every improvement you make inches the world forward by giving others an example to follow.

DAY 13: SHARPEN YOUR THINKING SKILLS

"(People) are apt to mistake the strength of their feeling for the
strength of their argument. The heated mind resents the chill
touch and relentless scrutiny of logic."
~ William E. Gladstone

Erica and I believe in *The Greek Ideal*, a harmonious blend of mind,
body, and spirit. Odysseus, the Greek hero from Homer's Odyssey,
was a mythological representation of the Greek ideal. During his 10-
year voyage from Troy back to Ithaca, Odysseus demonstrated
physical prowess, depth of character, and a sharp, clever intellect.
Odysseus was developed in all areas. The spokes of a wheel must be
balanced for the wheel to function best. By the same token, the life
domains of aging heroes must receive balanced development for our
lives to function best. When you think about improving yourself,
physical and emotional well-being are probably the first things that
come to mind. However, cognitive, or thinking skills, are as essential
to a full life as physical stamina and emotional stability.

Critical thinking skills are a sorely neglected aspect of personal
development. Critical thinking is "disciplined thinking that is clear,
rational, open-minded, and informed by evidence."[lxvi] The rewards
of honing critical thinking skills are mental clarity, sound
judgment, and protection from being played for a sucker. Someone
once said, "The mind, once stretched by a new idea, never returns
to its original dimensions."[lxvii] Critical thinking stretches the mind.
The difference between the mind of a critical thinker and the mind

of the average person is as pronounced as the difference between the physique of a bodybuilder and that of the average couch potato.

I have never met anyone who did not consider himself a critical thinker. However, if you have never been trained to think critically, the odds that you are a critical thinker are probably close to zero. Most people are what I call *natural thinkers*. Every animal on the planet navigates life by intuition or what *feels* right. *Natural thinkers*, people who have had no training in critical thinking, operate in the same way. Natural thinkers mistake feeling true for being true. If it is Tuesday, but it feels like it's Friday to me, it's still Tuesday. Feelings have no impact on facts.

If you ask someone what it would take to change their mind about a particular belief and they say, "nothing could change my mind," you know you are not talking to a critical thinker. Critical thinkers *are always willing to change their position when evidence indicates they are wrong*. This is what is meant by having an open mind. Being open-minded doesn't mean you are willing to entertain any and every crazy notion. It just means you are open to ideas that can be backed up with evidence and logic.

By nature, critical thinking leads to more questions than answers. For a skilled critical thinker, issues are seldom simple. Because critical thought requires approaching a problem from many angles, solutions tend to come in shades of gray rather than black and white. H.L. Menken wasn't far off the mark when he said, "For every complex problem, there is a simple solution… and it is always wrong."[lxviii] The primitive animal within us is highly attracted to simple solutions.

One of those simple solutions is to conform to your *ingroups* and be suspicious of your *outgroups*. Your ingroups are made up of the people you consider to be like you. Your outgroups are the people you see as being different from you. Treating the ingroups well and the outgroups poorly is a trait that is present all over the animal kingdom. The ingroup/outgroup thing happens between all social animals, from troops of monkeys to zeals of zebras.

Ingroup/outgroup is hardwired. Research has shown that even when people are randomly assigned to groups, they immediately consider their group better than the other groups! Ingroup/outgroup is the root cause of bigotry. Animal behaviors like ingroup/outgroup often dominate the lives of people who are not critical thinkers.

Conspiracy theories are fertile ground for working on thinking skills because everyone who has not been trained to think critically is vulnerable to believing them. Is global warming a hoax? Are pharmaceutical companies pushing harmful vaccines for profit? Is the world flat? Was the COVID-19 epidemic planned? Was 9/11 an inside job? Is the Earth only 5000 years old? Was the moon landing faked?

Why do the conspiracy theories we believe sound reasonable and the ones we don't believe sound foolish? These theories say much more about human nature than they do about reality. Which conspiracies you like will be affected by your politics, your religion, your culture, and your personality. *Believing a particular conspiracy theory in no way increases the likelihood that it is true.* Because they appeal to a paranoid vein in the human psyche, conspiracy theories exploit the fundamental human thinking error of *mistaking feeling true for being true.* Friedrich Nietzsche said, "There are two kinds of people in the world, those who want to know and those who want to believe."[lxix] Critical thinkers want to know. Conspiracy theorists want to believe.

Historically, conspiracy theorists were small, fringe groups who were ridiculed by the public. They were the weirdos in tinfoil hats hiding in their basements. Unfortunately, easy access to an avalanche of misinformation and an educational system that often omits critical thinking skills created a perfect storm for rising numbers of conspiracy theorists. Ideas that might have been recognized as ludicrous 20 years ago are given more respect by some than exhaustively researched scientific theories! Conspiracy theorists have emerged as a massive segment of mainstream society and have a powerful influence over national policy. The inmates are running the asylum! We can no longer ignore conspiracy theorists as a small group of kooks. Many people died because they believed conspiracy theories about the Covid-19 vaccines.

In the 12th century, William of Ockham gave us "Occam's Razor," a rule for cutting through bullshit information. In plain language, Occam's Razor says that the explanation with the fewest assumptions is usually correct. So, if I leave work and find that my tire is flat, various possibilities could explain what happened. Maybe a resentful student did the flattening. Perhaps the government is trying to make my life difficult. Maybe space aliens have been up to mischief. Or maybe I ran over a nail. Occam's Razor would steer me to the "ran over a nail" explanation. Occam's Razor would immediately replace most conspiracy theories with the answer provided by leading experts in whatever field the conspiracy theory addresses.

Critical thinkers are the opposite of conspiracy theorists. From a neutral place, critical thinkers weigh the quality and the quantity of the evidence from both sides of an argument to separate fact from fiction. *The facts that arise when you use critical thinking are seldom exciting and usually don't stroke your ego or validate your feelings.* If you are a critical thinker, finding the truth is more important than being right.

Following a logical chain of evidence usually shows most conspiracy theories to be, well, ridiculous. No one likes to be proven wrong, but critical thinkers prefer to be slightly embarrassed learners than self-satisfied fools. Replacing emotionally seductive but irrational ideas with reasonable ones may be uncomfortable, but it pays off with a clear understanding of the world around you.

While many critical thinkers are brilliant, a high IQ is not a requirement. Some intelligent people are very poor critical thinkers. Why? Because critical thinking is as much about emotions as it is about intellect. Changing your mind when the evidence dictates is the foundation of a developed mind. This goes against human nature. It doesn't *feel* good. It requires the wisdom to disregard the negative feelings associated with being proven wrong. Ironically, *learning is defined by moments of discovering that you are wrong.*

Conspiracy theorists believe in "evidence" that supports their theory no matter how flakey, and they discredit or ignore the evidence that disputes their theory no matter how solid. This is because the goal of the conspiracy theorist is not to find objective truth but to prove what they already believe. James Clear said, "Most people don't want accurate information. They want validating information. Growth requires you to be open to unlearn ideas that previously served you."[lxx]

The Dunning-Kruger effect shows the relationship between competence and confidence.[lxxi] Research shows that the less you know about a topic, the more confident you are that your opinion is correct. Pure ignorance yields maximum confidence. Bertrand Russell said, "the trouble with the world is that the stupid are cocksure and the intelligent are full of doubt."[lxxii] Charles Darwin made a similar comment, "ignorance more frequently begets confidence than knowledge."[lxxiii]

Years ago, when I earned my bachelor's degree, I remember naively considering myself an expert in psychology. Now, with a master's degree and 30-plus years of experience as an educator and practitioner, I recognize how little I know. Understanding the narrowness of my areas of expertise helps me accept my amateur status in nearly all other domains of knowledge. This gives me a profound respect for those who have committed the time and effort to become experts in their chosen fields. The car dealer I found in a chat room arguing with a medical doctor against the need for the Covid-19 vaccine is a living example of the Dunning-Kruger effect. Experts in every field have a breadth and depth of knowledge unknown to non-experts.

At this point in life, I find it hard to muster the arrogance to dispute NASA on space travel, the World Health Organization on medicine, or the World Meteorological Organization on climate. This is not to say that experts are always right, just that they are much more likely to be correct than those who are not experts. As adults have a much deeper understanding of life than children, experts have an exponentially deeper understanding of their areas of knowledge than novices.

Some guidelines for critical thinking:

1. High levels of certainty often mean low levels of critical thinking (consider talk radio hosts and New Age gurus).
2. Objective evidence and logic outweigh popular opinions and intuition.
3. "Feelings" are not evidence. "Common Sense" is not evidence. "Faith" is not evidence. "How I was raised" is not evidence. "Personal stories" are not evidence.
4. Changing positions when opposing evidence outweighs supporting evidence is the hallmark of critical thought.
5. Ego is the greatest hindrance to critical thinking.

NOTEBOOK ACTIVITY: TRUST THE EXPERTS

Write down the conspiracy theories that you are attracted to, then research what the consensus of experts says on the subject.

For example, if I am attracted to the global warming conspiracy, I would search, *"What do the majority of experts think about the global warming conspiracy?"*

The first answer I found when I did this search was from Wikipedia:

"A 2019 review of scientific papers found the consensus on the cause of climate change to be at 100%, and a 2021 study concluded that over

99% of scientific papers agree on the human cause of climate change. Papers that disagreed with the consensus either cannot be replicated or contain errors."

Becoming a critical thinker requires courage and maturity. It takes guts because it will sometimes mean going against ideas you grew up with and ideas that are popular with your friends and family. It takes maturity because immature people are generally incapable of overriding their gut feelings. Courage and maturity are also defining characteristics of aging heroes!

BEING A SPIRITUAL HERO

"You have to know what sparks the light in you so that you, in your own way, can illuminate the world."[lxxiv]
~ Oprah Winfrey

In his book, "Spirituality: A Brief History,"[lxxv] Phillip Sheldrake defines spirituality as "the deepest values and meanings by which people live." So, a spiritual person remains centered on her code of honor and her personal philosophy. Maintaining that center can be a challenge. A world of intruding forces competes for your attention to throw you off your mark. Spiritual practices can restore you to your purpose and help you to stay on point even when life sends you a tempest.

DAY 14: EXPERIENCE WONDER

"The mind is not a vessel to be filled, but a fire to be kindled."[lxxvi]
~ Plutarch

The opportunity to live a human life is a miraculous gift. Look around you. Notice the beauty in your environment. As children, we are in awe of even the simplest phenomena. Children are fascinated by the textured bark on a tree, the sound of the breeze rustling leaves, and the fragrance of a wildflower. That sense of endless wonder can fade as we age. In adulthood, our minds are so focused on daily responsibilities that we become blind and deaf to the magic of the universe around us.

Consider this. The objects you encounter in a dream seem to have similar physical properties to objects in real life. You experience them as having weight, color, and form, but they are made from nothing. As scientists delved deeper and deeper into what makes up solid matter in the real world, they found that matter is composed of molecules, that are composed of atoms, and atoms are composed of 99.999999999999 percent empty space.[lxxvii] At the most negligible levels, matter is made from almost nothing. What you experience in real life is as much a simulation created by your brain as what you experience when you are dreaming!

Every physical property, sight, sound, smell, and texture only exists in relation to someone experiencing them. If a tree falls in the woods and there is no one there to hear it, does it make a sound? This may take a bit of mental stretching, but the answer is "No." Sound is a relationship between a phenomenon in the environment (vibrations), an ear, and a brain. If one part of the relationship is missing, sound cannot happen. Visual images are the same. An image is a relationship between something in the environment (reflected light), an eye, and a brain. No eye or brain? No image. Your living in what seems to be a physical world composed of solid matter is magical. You give the universe form and substance! It comes into being every time you open your eyes and ears to experience it. You are the universe experiencing itself. Grasp the awe of that!

How about this? Life began on our planet 3.8 billion years ago. Large numbers like a billion are impossible for humans to conceptualize. Close your eyes and create a mental image of 5 randomly organized beach balls. Not too difficult, right? Now close your eyes and try to create an accurate image of 100 beach balls. An accurate mental image of 100 randomly organized beach balls is impossible. It just looks like a lot of beach balls. Now try 1000 beach balls. My mental picture of 1000 beach balls looks just like my image of a million, billion, or trillion beach balls. Suffice it to say that 3.8 billion is an incomprehensible amount of time. Millions and millions of generations of life forms evolved in tiny increments from one-celled organisms to the incredible range of diverse life forms that currently inhabit the planet. In this vast ocean of space, time, and life emerges YOU! The odds of you being alive in this time and place are astronomically small. Your existence is a miracle!

Recapturing your sense of wonder can be a satisfying way to enrich your life. Experiencing awe is transformative. It sharpens your mind and sparks creativity. It decreases stress and improves immunity. Wonder is free and highlights appreciation for experiences rather than possessions. Wonder moves you into a flow state. Flow has been described as "the holistic sensation that people feel when they act with total involvement."[lxxviii] Awe removes your *self* from the equation, and everything merges into the experience. As this happens, you have a better sense of your connection with others and have an increased desire to assist them in improving their lives.

Here are some ideas on how to reignite that lost sense of wonder:

- *Follow your curiosity.* Children are endlessly curious, and experience wonder regularly. The world will always be a wonder when you take the time to explore those things you are curious about. Ask questions and seek answers. Especially enjoy those questions that don't have definite answers.

- *Try thought experiments.* Go online and search for thought experiments. Erica and I find them fascinating. They are fun and have the potential to help you generate new insights about life. Here is one of our favorites created by John Rawls: *Suppose you and a group of people had to decide on the principles to establish a new society. However, none of you know anything about who you will be in that society. Your race, income level, sex, gender, religion, and personal preferences are all unknown to you. After you decide on those principles, you will be turned out into the society you established.* [lxxix]

- *Embrace diversity.* Visit new places. Befriend people who are different from you. Explore art, music, cuisine, religions, geographies, and languages unfamiliar to you.

- *Have deep conversations.* Find people who are captivated by ideas and engage them. The minds of other thinkers are infinitely intriguing.

- *Be here now.* Allow the social mask you wear to crumble and fall away. What is beneath is pure beauty. Take a moment to be without concern about being judged by others. Singing, dancing, and playing music often help Erica and me lose ourselves and take us to the space of wonder.

NOTEBOOK ACTIVITY: IMMERSE YOURSELF IN WONDER

Set aside a few minutes each day to dwell in the space of wonder. Allow your natural curiosity to guide you. Use the suggestions herein or devise your own creative way to find awe. Describe your experiences in your notebook. Make experiencing wonder a life habit.

DAY 15: MEDITATE

"When you're a kid, you lay in the grass and watch the clouds going over, and you don't have a thought in your mind. It's purely meditation, and we lose that."[lxxx]
~ Dick Van Dyke

I have heard sailing described as ninety percent boring and ten percent terrifying. I'm afraid I have to disagree with that. I think sailing is ninety percent *meditative* and ten percent terrifying! Meditation isn't strange or mystical and doesn't have to be religious. Humans and animals meditate all the time naturally. Our Labrador retriever, Keel, spends much of his time in a meditative state. He lays there for long periods, relaxed, sometimes with his eyes open, sometimes with his eyes closed, but he is not asleep. If a dog barks in the neighborhood, a car door slams shut, or someone walks up the front steps, he springs to his feet perfectly alert. When Keel is sleeping, he is slow to awaken and generally needs a good stretch before he gets going.

Have you ever driven on a long trip alone without a radio? If so, you may have found yourself so lost in thought that time passed without your awareness. You may have thought to yourself, "Who has been driving for the past two hours?!" This is an example of a meditative experience. Any extended, uninterrupted, repetitive behavior will likely create a meditative state. Knitting, mowing the lawn, weeding a garden, operating a tractor, and even washing dishes or folding laundry can all trigger meditative, *self-transcendent flow states*.

Self-transcendence is a shift from the typical conscious state of *duality* to one of *flow*. Duality comes from the word *dual,* which just means two. In ordinary consciousness, you experience two things, you and everything that is not you. Self-transcendence means switching from experiencing you in relation to all other things to a state where everything merges into the flow of experience. You disappear into the experience. Instead of you knitting, there is just *knitting*. Instead of you weeding, there is just *weeding*.

When you first learned to drive a car, you were keenly aware of yourself in relation to the many actions and objects involved in the process of driving. There was you in relation to the gas pedal. You in relation to the steering wheel. You in relation to the other cars on the road. You in relation to the traffic lights. However, once you became an experienced driver and took that long trip without the radio, you faded into the experience of driving. Instead of *you* driving the *car*, there was just *driving. You* and your *experience* were no longer separate. You were self-transcendent.

The stress response is the most extreme experience of duality. Stress is when the *self* feels threatened by something that is *not the self*. It is the polar opposite of the self-transcendent flow state that occurs in meditation. So, it should not be surprising that meditation is an effective tool for combating all emotional, cognitive, and physical health problems caused by stress.[lxxxi] Meditation is a proven stress reducer with numerous emotional and physical health benefits. Meditation has been found to decrease anxiety, even in people with clinical anxiety disorders. It improves attention and concentration while enhancing self-awareness by helping you better understand your thought and behavior processes. Meditation can improve memory, relieve depression and anxiety, slow down the aging process, decrease cardiovascular disease, decrease obesity, decrease diabetes, and it may even extend life![lxxxii lxxxiii lxxxiv]

In one experiment, meditators and non-meditators were connected to biofeedback equipment and shown a typical action movie. As the excitement in the film reached its crescendo, both groups showed signs of fight-or-flight arousal. Heart rates increased, blood pressures increased, sweating increased, etcetera. The differences came when the exciting peak of the movie was over. When the excitement ended, the meditators' bio signs returned to normal, while the non-meditators remained aroused. Meditation connected its practitioners to the present moment, allowing their fight-or-flight responses to operate healthily.

NOTEBOOK ACTIVITY: YOUR MEDITATION EXPERIENCES

Write down a few times when you have unknowingly entered a meditative state. What were these experiences like? Can you think of times in your life when you experienced a self-transcendent flow state? Have you ever disappeared into your experience, and time passed without your awareness?

DAY 16: CENTER YOURSELF

"To meditate means to go home to yourself. Then you know how to take care of the things that are happening inside you, and you know how to take care of the things that happen around you."[lxxxv]
~ Thich Nhat Hanh

Success in meditation has nothing to do with feelings of accomplishment. Sitting meditation is like no other activity on earth. It is the opposite of doing something. Success in meditation does not mean having a magical experience. It does not mean becoming blissful or enlightened. Success in meditation is the act of practicing. If you practice and feel like nothing happened, you have still succeeded. If you practice every day for a month and feel like nothing has happened, you have still succeeded. Practice *is* a success.

Meditation is not an inactive mental state. It requires sustained focused attention. Research has shown that brain structures are transformed through meditation.[lxxxvi] Among other changes, people who meditate regularly have been found to have a thickening of the prefrontal cortex, the area of the brain that governs attention, concentration, and executive functions (decision-making). Regular meditation improves mental and emotional fitness.

There are many schools of meditation. For aging heroes, we recommend two meditation strategies, 1) sitting meditation and 2) mindfulness meditation. Below are instructions on how to add sitting meditation into your wellness lifestyle:

SITTING MEDITATION

1. Clear your schedule for uninterrupted meditation.
2. Choose a space for your practice. Make it comfortable and private.
3. Music with long slow notes played at a low volume can help to calm the mind's chatter. New Age Spa music is perfect for this.
4. Set an alarm for how long you plan to practice so you don't need to check the time. Start with something easy, 5 minutes, and work your way up to a daily 20-minute session.
5. Find a comfortable position. Some people lie down to meditate. I prefer to sit. Lying down can make me sleepy; meditation is about focused attention. Erica likes to lie down to meditate. She doesn't have my drowsiness issue.
6. Take three of four slow, deep breaths, in through the nose and out through the mouth. Slow, controlled breathing can slow your heart rate, decrease blood pressure, and relax you.
7. Create an image in your mind that represents the Aging Hero. The defining characteristics of heroes are honor, courage, and conviction. Now, imagine *yourself* as the embodiment of these qualities. Fill in the details. How does it feel inside to be that Aging Hero? What expression do you have on your face? What does your posture look like? Burn that image into your mind and hold it there.
8. As you breathe deeply and slowly, try to keep your mind focused on the image you created.
    a. Your mind may wander (a lot). Each time it does, gently bring your attention back to the image of yourself as the personification of the Aging Hero. If you must bring your mind back 1000 times, you are still meditating successfully.
    b. Allow distracting thoughts to flare and disappear like sparks.

    c. Meditation is not about beating your mind into submission. It is about patiently refocusing your attention in a kind and gentle manner.

9. Stay put until your alarm sounds.

One meditation life hack that Erica and I use is the *Insight Timer* meditation app. Insight Timer is the most comprehensive meditation app we have found. People all over the world use it to improve sleep and decrease stress and anxiety. Erica also uses the *Calm app* to help manage stress.

NOTEBOOK ACTIVITY: MEDITATE

Try a five-minute meditation using the nine steps above and write down a brief description of your experience. Was it boring? Was it frustrating? Was it relaxing? Regardless of your experience, you were successful if you followed the steps. Congrats!

Buddhists compare the mind to a wild monkey that tears around uncontrolled. Note the many ways your monkey mind rebels against the practice of meditation. The more you practice, the more you can control your mind. The monkey runs the show in an untrained mind, and it leads you around by the nose. Meditation puts you in charge of the monkey rather than the other way around. Sitting meditation shines a bright light on your relationship with yourself.

DAY 17: BE MINDFUL

"With mindfulness, you can establish yourself in the present to touch the wonders of life that are available in that moment."[lxxxvii]
~ Thich Nhat Hanh

Mindfulness is pretty much what it sounds like. It is the practice of being mindful in daily life. In sitting meditation, you choose a single item to focus on. In mindfulness meditation, your life is the object of focus. Considering the fantastic opportunity we have each been given to live exactly one human life, most of us allow much of the experience to pass without our notice. While brushing our teeth in the morning, we are preoccupied with planning our day. While driving to work, we are thinking about our to-do list. While doing our work, we daydream about going home. Once home, we stress about tomorrow's work.

Our minds are forever dreaming about the future or ruminating over the past. The truth is, neither the future nor the past is real. All we ever have is the present. Given that the present is where we will live our entire lives, doesn't it make sense to drink in the experience for all it is worth?

Mindfulness is the act of gently bringing your mind back from inner processes to the only place you will ever reside, the here and now. Being mindful of the sights, smells, sounds, flavors, tactile (touch), and kinesthetic (movement) sensations of this present moment makes life richer and more textured because nothing is wasted. Being present is being genuinely alive rather than simply thinking about living. Mindfulness and wellness are two sides of the same coin.

In life, there are peaks, valleys, and plateaus.[lxxxviii] The peaks are the things we look forward to. Graduation, getting married, going on vacation, and getting that promotion are "peak" experiences. Losing a loved one, getting sick, and having disappointments are "valley" experiences. Daily activities like getting dressed, checking the mail, cleaning your house, and taking a shower are usually "plateau" experiences. In varying degrees, all of our lives will have peaks. All will have valleys. And, all will have plateaus. If life were a pie, peaks and valleys would be slivers, and the rest of the pie would be the plateaus! Now, consider the inordinate amount of time the average person spends thinking about the peaks and valleys compared to the time they spend paying attention to the plateaus. What a waste! It is like ignoring the pleasure of eating a delicious, four-course meal by being preoccupied with dessert.

Much of life is spent in the daily grind, the plateau. We get up, get dressed, cook, clean, drive, do chores, and go to work day after day. We find many of these activities boring or unpleasant. I used to hate washing dishes until I learned about mindfulness. Instead of dreading and grumbling through this daily chore, I deactivated the negative emotions connected with washing dishes by genuinely experiencing the process.

I turn on the water and listen to the sound as it runs into the sink. It is pleasant. I put my hands under the pouring water and enjoy the cool flow as it gradually becomes warm. I add dish soap, and the scent of lemon fills the air as a pile of bubbles grows. I pick up the sponge and attend to the texture against my hands and fingers. I wash the first plate and notice its smoothness. I watch as the dish changes from dirty to clean and feel a sense of satisfaction. I rinse it, place the dish on the rack, and appreciate how it balances there.

Mindfulness changed my most dreaded daily activity from a drudgery to a profoundly vivid experience. *Every one of life's daily activities can be made expansive through mindfulness. Every relationship can be made deeper through mindfulness.* If you have ever had a friend, loved one, or therapist genuinely listen to you instead of waiting for their turn to talk, you know what a gift it is. That listener was practicing mindfulness. Mindful listening strengthens the bonds people have with each other.

Some people are naturally more mindful than others, but all of us can improve. In sitting meditation, the process is to gently return your mind to the object of your meditative focus (perhaps the image of yourself as an iconic Aging Hero). Mindfulness is the constant process of gently refocusing attention back to the sensations of this present moment.

MINDFULNESS MEDITATION

Mindfulness should be an ongoing practice. You should, of course, enjoy fantasy, planning, and creative thinking whenever you like. But, during your daily activities, try practicing mindfulness at every opportunity:

1. Slow down and zero in on the pleasures that can be gleaned from ordinary life. Allow yourself to smile frequently.
2. Use *child's mind*, a Buddhist concept for experiencing the world with fresh eyes as a child would. Think of a young child's fascination with something as simple as examining a feather.
3. Gently remind yourself to be here now at every opportunity. Use external signals as reminders to re-engage mindfulness.
4. You can use traffic lights, opening doors, doorbells, mealtime, walking from one room to another, the ringing of a phone, standing up, sitting down, or any other frequent occurrences as triggers to remind you to come back to the present.
5. Appreciate the subtle sensory experiences of living.
6. In your interactions with others, be present and truly listen to them.

7. Do not get frustrated with yourself. The object is to find joy in simple experiences. Redirecting yourself back to the present moment ten thousand times is a success, not a failure.

NOTEBOOK ACTIVITY: PRACTICE MINDFULNESS

For the rest of the day, use the steps above to practice mindfulness whenever you think about it. Jot down your insights. Make mindfulness a priority in your life. You only live once. Might as well be there for it!

DAY 18: FIND ADVENTURE

"We live in a wonderful world that is full of beauty, charm, and adventure. There is no end to the adventures that we can have if only we seek them with our eyes open."[lxxxix]
~ Jawaharlal Nehru

Adventure keeps the spirit alive! It occurs anytime you experience excitement and risk. The choice to be an aging hero is inherently adventurous. Aging heroes do not conform to society's expectations. This means we risk rejection from small-minded people leading what Henry David Thoreau called "lives of quiet desperation."[xc] Such folks are imprisoned by the limitations placed on them by others, and they resent all who have set themselves free. Jack Nicholson's character in the movie *Easy Rider* describes this well, "They'll talk to ya and talk to ya and talk to ya about individual freedom. But if they see a free individual, it's gonna scare 'em."[xci] Fear and anger are manifestations of the fight or flight response. They emerge whenever people feel threatened. By nature, free people often fail to conform. This can be pretty threatening to some folks.

On the other hand, some yearn to be free from society's constraints but lack the wherewithal to break away. Those people will admire your courage and may even be inspired to become aging heroes themselves! Being your authentic self tends to magnetize the types of people you want in your life and repel people who would bring you down.

Erica and I enjoy adventures, great and small. She once did a 24-hour relay race across one of the Hawaiian islands. She traveled in a van with a group of 6 participants who took turns running day and night from Hilo to Kona. The van would drop a runner off at a checkpoint and then drive to the next checkpoint. At the next checkpoint, a new runner would exit the van to run her leg of the race. The route went through multiple climates, from hot and dry, to wet and cold. And from deserts to mountains to beaches. Erica tells stories of running through a volcanic desert at 2 am. What an adventure!

I was a member of a full-patch motorcycle club, or MC, for a year. The full patch is a big deal in the biker community because any club wishing to sport one must get permission to do so from the dominant *one-percenter* club. One-percenter motorcycle clubs are also called *outlaw* clubs. The U.S. Department of Justice considers outlaw clubs criminal enterprises.[xcii] Examples of one-percenter clubs are the Hell's Angels, the Pagans, the Outlaws, and the Banditos. Each area in the US has a dominant one-percenter club. Failure to go through the process of getting permission to use a full patch can result in violent enforcement. The club I belonged to was not a one-percenter club, but my club refused to ask permission to wear the full patch. This put us at risk any time my club members wore their *cuts*, the vests with the identifying club patches on the back. Conflicts between my club and one-percenter clubs occurred, but I was never involved in one. The whole thing sounds silly, but it is deadly serious for club guys.

My biker name was "The Professor." The handle stuck. I had a lot of fun and took a lot of risks as an MC member. A hundred of us would ride two abreast, so close that I could reach out and touch the handlebar of the rider beside me. There would be about a foot of space between the bikes in front and behind me. We rode in this formation at crazy speeds for 50 miles at a clip. It was supposed to be an exercise in trust. If anyone in the group were to make a mistake, it would have wiped out the string of bikers traveling behind. The biker club lifestyle was ultimately not for me, but I had plenty of adventure during my tenure.

Erica and I live in the mountains of Western North Carolina, where there are many opportunities for outdoor adventure. Sailing, kayaking, backpacking, hiking, white-water rafting, geocaching, and dragon boat racing are all activities at our doorstep. Many of these pastimes are either cheap or free. Every geographical region offers unique opportunities for adventure. What is available in your area?

Adventures are not limited to physical challenges. Adventures happen every time you move out of your comfort zone. You can have adventures by experiencing movies, music, and literature that are not from your preferred genres. You may enjoy spiritual adventures by exploring new philosophical and religious practices and perspectives. You can have adventures of the mind by following your curiosity and exploring new ideas.

You can have social adventures by making friends with people who are different from you or culinary adventures by trying exotic foods. When it comes to diversity and inclusion, our culture is still in its infancy. These issues are usually framed as they relate to fairness and morality. What is often left out of the discussion is that increasing diversity and inclusion is fun and interesting! Interacting with people from different cultures is a fascinating way to broaden your horizons. Variety is the spice of life. Erica and I are an interracial couple. We are endlessly intrigued by each other's cultural perspectives. Our relationship is an adventure.

At this stage of life, you have no doubt noticed how much the passage of time seems to speed up as you age. I first became aware of this the year I finished college. High school seemed to last a lifetime, but college was over before I could blink twice. The time that has passed since college has felt like half a blink. One theory about this phenomenon involves having fewer novel or unique experiences as you age.[xciii] As a young child, everything is new to you. Every day brings new knowledge and new experiences. As you age, the number of novel experiences begins to decrease. If you are not careful, your life can become monotonous. The same morning routine. The same work routine. The same recreation routine. Monotony does not afford opportunities for creating new memories. New memories are one way we mark the passage of time. Without new experiences to file away, time seems to pass very rapidly. Social, emotional, physical, and spiritual diversity makes your life interesting, allows you to create new memories, and slows down your perception of the passage of time. Mindfulness is a way of noticing subtle changes in your environment. This process transforms everyday experiences into novel ones and has the effect of making time more expansive.

I was always interested in travel, but I did not make it a priority. I never felt I had the finances to go abroad. Spending money on experiences seemed frivolous and unnecessary to me. As a result, I didn't leave the US until I was 50. Meanwhile, before we knew each other, Erica was globe-trotting all over Europe. How did she do it? She wasn't any more financially secure than I was. Erica prioritized experiences over possessions. She knew intuitively what research has now shown to be a key to life satisfaction. Experiences bring greater and more lasting joy than material things.[xciv] Psychologists found that buying *experiences* (like travel, entertainment, outdoor activities, and eating out) delivered more happiness before, during, and after the purchase than buying *things* (like clothes, jewelry, electronics, and furniture).[xcv]

Think about what happens after you buy an item you want. Imagine something big, a new car. You buy a new car and feel great happiness for a few days, but your joy is temporary. You begin to see people with better and newer cars than yours. Before long, your car becomes just another car, and the joy it brought you is forgotten. Now imagine instead that you take a trip to explore the jungles of Costa Rica. You feel happiness planning the trip. You feel pleasure during the trip. And you feel happy for the rest of your life whenever you share stories about the trip with others.

At a party, would you be more interested in hanging out with the person who is talking about her new car or the person who is telling the story of her adventures in the Costa Rican jungles? Your experiences, not your things, make you who you are. In a very real way, experiences define you. Human beings are social creatures. We are hardwired with a need to connect with others. Experiences can enhance social connections. Material things typically can not. Erica and I are not wealthy people, but when it comes to spending, we prioritize experiences over things. This even affects the gifts we buy for loved ones. We are much more likely to give someone a gift certificate for an hour-massage than a new sweater. Life satisfaction is about *being* and *doing*, not about *having*.

I have always been a dreamer. My teachers in grade school used to write that on my report cards! As an adult, I often fantasize about my bucket list but then drop the ball before ever making anything happen. In daily life, I get things done, but when it comes to big purchases, I have a hard time pulling the trigger. Erica is *great* at pulling that particular trigger. In my mid-fifties, I told Erica I wanted to learn to sail. I grew up on the coast, but we always had motorboats. The thought of moving across the water, harnessing the wind as people have done for thousands of years, lit me up. The idea would have ended as a pipe dream if Erica hadn't pushed for buying a sailboat.

Sailing has its own language and its own culture. I compare it to playing the guitar. It is not difficult to learn to strum a song or two on the guitar, and it is not hard to learn to take a sailboat out for a spin. However, learning to be a good guitarist or a true sailor takes years of practice. The time we have spent sailing and learning about sailing has created some of our best memories. Sailing is one of our favorite adventurous activities. Where do you find adventure in your life?

NOTEBOOK ACTIVITY: MAKE AN ADVENTURE BUCKET LIST

Write down a few adventures you would like to have over the next year. They can be small adventures like trying exotic food from another country or big adventures like skydiving. Set a date and follow through on them as soon as possible. What obstacles might prevent you from making those things happen (indecisiveness, finances, health, time, fear)? How can you overcome these barriers? My goals before I turned 60 were to run a marathon and to learn to surf. We registered for a race and immediately started training. Covid ended our training and caused the race to be canceled, but we got up to 18 miles in training runs. I didn't reach my goal, but I did compete in a half-marathon. I still file it away as a win. How many other 60-year-olds with lung disease can say they ran 18 miles? I am not ruling out another marathon goal for the future. That year, we also traveled to Bocas Del Toro, Panama, a major surfing destination. Erica signed us up for surfing lessons, and we hit the beaches. Make your adventures happen. There's no time to waste!

DAY 19: CREATE YOUR CODE OF HONOR

"Honor is simply the morality of superior people."
~ H. L. Mencken

Another aspect of spirituality is morality. Greek heroes, samurai warriors, knights of old, religious groups, people in the armed services, and even girl scouts and boy scouts have codes of honor. A code of honor is a set of rules for moral behavior. All animals will try to avoid harm. Even an amoeba will move away from an electric shock. Amoebas don't need a code of honor, only self-preservation. Unlike amoebas, humans are social animals. In nature, ancient humans required the help of other humans to survive. For people, self-preservation went along with the preservation of *the tribe*. Moral rules grew from human dependence on one another. Other social animals like buffalo and lions will sometimes behave in ways that promote the health and safety of the group over the health and safety of one individual. However, only humans create moral codes to live by.

Morality quickly becomes a part of who we are. So much so that it feels like we were born with it. We were not. Babies have no morals. They scream and cry with complete disregard for how it affects other people. Morality is a learned behavior. Feral children who have not been exposed to other humans have three things in common.[xcvi] They don't walk. They don't talk. And they don't have a sense of morality. There are critical periods in a child's development during which they are primed for learning specific skills. If the child does not acquire those skills during that critical window of time, she will likely never fully develop them. Think of how easy it is for a small child to learn a language and how difficult it is to learn a new language in adulthood. The critical developmental window for learning language is during early childhood. Feral children who are rescued from isolation can never fully develop a moral sense because the critical developmental window for learning morality has closed.

There are three levels of moral development.[xcvii]

Level 1: We begin socializing young children by rewarding "good" behaviors and punishing "bad" ones. The moral rules that determine good and bad will come from external sources like parents, teachers, religious texts, and laws. At first, children will follow the rules whenever an authority figure is watching, but they will break the rules when they think there will be no consequences. My dog is at this level of moral development. He knows he will be in trouble if he gets into the trash. When Erica and I are around, he never breaks the trash rule, but when we leave him home alone, he knocks over the damn trash can every time. The slogan for the first level of moral development is, "What's in it for me?" Human adults who stay at this first level of moral development are sociopaths with no regard for others. For them, other people are there to be used for personal gain.

Level 2: Older children internalize the rules they learned from their caregivers. They start to self-regulate by trying to do the right thing even when no one else is around. They do this because they want to be "good boys and girls." They want approval from the authority figures in their lives. Most people stay at this level of moral development for life. They learned the rules for moral behavior from their culture. Their parents, ministers, police officers, teachers, schools, churches, and courts all reinforced the rules of their culture.

People at this second level of morality try to follow the rules they learned. The end.

So, what's wrong with that? The problem is that we were not all raised by the same parents, in the same cultures, or with the same religions and laws. For centuries, people have fought and killed each other over who has the correct moral code. In the same way that you are confident that *you* have true morality, every other person on Earth has the same certainty that *they* have true morality. People raised by Nazis are as sure in their righteousness as people raised by saints. Our egos assure each of us that we happened to hit the magic jackpot to be raised with the one true moral code.

If you were a white person raised in the Southern United States in the early 1800s, chances are your parents, ministers, police officers, teachers, schools, churches, and courts would all have reinforced the idea that slavery was ok. Slavery had been around for thousands of years. In the Bible, the word slavery refers both to slavery in the traditional sense and what we would call indentured servitude. The Bible instructs people on how to treat their slaves but never indicates that slavery is wrong. In the same way some modern ministers currently use the Bible to justify homophobia, some ministers in the 1800s used the Bible to justify slavery.[xcviii] If you were in the second stage of moral development and your culture determined your moral code, how would you know that slavery was wrong? You wouldn't. For that, you would need to move to the highest level of moral development.

Level 3: In the final stage of moral development, you take the moral code you learned from your culture and question it. For every moral issue, ask three questions. They represent universal moral litmuses:

Is harm done?
Is it fair?
Would I want me or someone I love to be treated like this?

By asking these three questions, you could determine that slavery is immoral regardless of where or when you were raised.

Does slavery do harm? Yep

Is slavery fair? Nope

Would I want me or someone I love to be treated like a slave? No way

"That's just how I was raised" is a lame excuse to behave immorally. As a child, you had no control over the moral ideas you learned. As an adult, you are responsible for examining moral beliefs and determining their actual value. As with every aspect of life, aging heroes choose a code of honor that transcends the status quo. We stand for what is right even when it conflicts with the cultures we grew up in. Create your own code of honor. Cull through the beliefs you grew up with and ask the three questions. The values you were raised with always feel true initially but feeling true and being true are not always the same. Level 2 morality is easy. It just means doing what you are told without question. Level 3 morality takes mad courage to execute because it often means going against the tide of the culture in which you were raised. Robert Kennedy said, "Few… are willing to brave the disapproval of their fellows… the wrath of society. Moral courage is a rarer commodity than bravery in battle or great intelligence. Yet, it is the one essential, vital quality for those who seek to change the world."[xcix]

This courage to go against the grain is the stuff of true heroes. Howard Zinn said, "Historically, the most terrible things, war, genocide, and slavery, have resulted not from disobedience, but from obedience."[c] Level 3 morality sometimes means being disobedient. Heroic actions all include risk. Some of the greatest heroes in history suffered horribly for standing up for values that represented genuine morality by showing disobedience to the false morality embraced by society.

NOTEBOOK ACTIVITY: YOUR CODE OF HONOR

Write down your code of honor. What are your rules to live by regarding how you treat your fellow human beings? Are there values you grew up with that don't hold up to the three questions? I was raised in a culture with a lot of overt bigotry. I am grateful to have developed a code of honor that is fair, does no harm, and comes from a place of empathy.

DAY 20: BE CREATIVE

"Creativity is arguably our most uniquely human trait. It enables us to escape the present, reconstruct the past, and fantasize about the future, to visualize something that does not exist and change the world with it."[ci]

~ Liane Gabora

Some people are naturally more creative than others. However, we all have the potential for creativity. Creativity is the ability to come up with and utilize unusual ideas. Creativity is at the core of the Aging Heroes lifestyle. The cookie-cutter solutions society provides us are the recipe for mediocrity. When life offers us a paint-by-numbers package, aging heroes paint outside the lines and off the canvas using colors not found in the kit. Creating meaning is our primary purpose and what that might look like is as varied and unique as each creator.

I knew a guy who was a sad example of someone who never took the opportunity to create meaning. If you read George Orwell's Animal Farm, he was Boxer, the horse. He lived by society's definition of what he should be and never questioned it. He was an earner and a consumer. He was honest, hard-working, and followed all the rules. This fellow was motivated by earning, but the other aspects of his life received less attention. As a father and husband, he was often absent due to work travel.

This guy used to spend hours and hours tallying up figures for future earnings. It was one of his favorite pastimes. He always talked about how in 5 more years, he was going to be "sitting pretty." Five more years, then five more years, then five more years. He never got to sit pretty. He just died. He never took the risk of trying to be creative. He had considered such an effort a waste of time. He never wrote a poem, drew a picture, wrote a love letter, or built a birdhouse. His lifelong commitment to earning and consuming was never rewarded. He left nothing of himself behind to mark his time on earth. Those who buy into society's philosophy of life, that meaning comes only from earning and spending, are destined to be treated as so much firewood, burned, forgotten, and replaced.

It takes creativity to design a meaningful life, but invention, for its own sake, can also be of great value. Creative people bring things into being that would not otherwise exist. Every song, painting, sculpture, poem, or handmade clay pot you create is an enduring part of you that might bring joy and meaning to others long after you are gone.

There are so many benefits to creativity. Creativity tends to relate to higher levels of emotional intelligence or EQ.[cii] Emotional intelligence is your ability to regulate and communicate your own emotions and to understand the feelings of others. Despite the stereotype of the tortured artist, positive moods result in increased creativity.[ciii] What's more, the reverse is also true. The more people engage in creative activities, the more they feel happy and flourishing.[civ] Negative and neutral moods don't affect creativity one way or the other. Creativity is also closely related to academic success.[cv] Generally speaking, creative people do better in school.

Often, people who do not have the wherewithal to create something will be the first to put down the creations of others. Adam Grant said, "Criticizing is easy and fast. Creating is difficult and slow. The two hours you spent on a book or a movie usually took two years to produce. Anyone can tear down someone else's work. The true test of insight is whether you can help them make it better or build something of your own."[cvi]

So how do you do it? If you don't consider yourself particularly creative, here are some tips that might help:

1. Expose yourself to new ideas. Creative ideas tend to spawn more creative ideas. I love checking out science and psychology podcasts because I am fascinated by unique ideas. One of my favorite pastimes is exploring ideas with Erica.

2. Practice thinking outside of the box by brainstorming. Try to come up with as many possible uses as you can think of for a brick. The uses don't have to be practical. The goal is to generate new ideas.

3. Spend time alone without distractions. Some of my most creative ideas came when I drove alone on a trip with the radio off. The mind is sometimes triggered to become creative in the void of boredom.

4. Play creative games. Pictionary, charades, Cranium, role play, and even hide-and-seek all require creative thought.

5. Learn a new language. Languages influence how people think. Learning a new language can treat you to a new way of understanding the world.

6. Keep a dream journal and a daydream journal. Crazy, engaging, and unique ideas flow from the unconscious when you dream. Freud called dreams "the royal road to the unconscious."[cvii] Daydreams are another source of creativity. Make time to daydream and allow your thoughts to flow. You'll be surprised by what you find.

7. Work on your mood. Research has shown that people are more creative when they are in a good mood and more analytical when they are in a bad mood. Gratitude, mindfulness, exercise, and getting good sleep are all factors that contribute to a good mood and hence, improved creativity.[cviii]

NOTEBOOK ACTIVITY: BE CREATIVE

Do one creative act and write it down. You may be an extremely creative person or feel that you don't have a creative bone in your body. If you have been doing the notebook activities in this book, you have already done a great deal of creating. Do one more. Write a poem. Draw a picture. Write a song. Make up a new recipe. Anything you come up with will count. Then, write about what it felt like to engage in creativity.

BEING A SOCIAL HERO

"I define connection as the energy that exists between people when they feel seen, heard, and valued; when they can give and receive without judgment; and when they derive sustenance and strength from the relationship."[cix]
~ Brené Brown

We are social by nature. Primitive humans could not survive without each other. Pound for pound, we are the weakest animals on the planet. Socially successful cave people who worked together remained in the gene pool, while social failures were culled out.

Among modern humans, some of us are extroverts who tend to be energized by social interactions, and some of us are introverts and need to recharge after social engagements. As an extrovert, I enjoy a beautiful sunset much more if I have someone to share the experience with. Erica is an introvert and says that a beautiful sunset is just as meaningful for her whether she is alone or with someone else. When she is by herself, she considers such experiences as unique gifts just for her. Regardless of our introvert/extrovert orientations, we all need connections with other people.

Our social connections help to define us and give our lives meaning. In some ways, the value of our relative social pools is outside our awareness. Like a fish that doesn't notice the ocean until it is removed from the water, we don't realize the importance of our social network until it is damaged or lost.

DAY 21: DO ROMANTIC RELATIONSHIPS RIGHT

"The good life is built with good relationships."
~ Robert J. Waldinger

Ever wonder why some couples seem to have it together? How do they pull that off? Wellness and healthy relationships go hand in hand. After many years of stumbling blindly (and largely unsuccessfully) through romantic relationships, I was lucky to connect with my incredible wife, Erica. She is smart, kind, sensitive, caring, creative, flexible, thoughtful, insightful, beautiful, and motivated. The fact that Erica rocks doesn't hurt, but her awesomeness does not account for the success of our relationship. She, like me, went through a long series of failed relationships before we connected. We frequently talk about our good fortune in finding one another and what makes our relationship work so well. Here are some of our insights:

WE ACCEPTED RESPONSIBILITY FOR PAST RELATIONSHIP FAILURES.

Erica and I got together late in life. We both had vowed never to marry again. Multiple failed marriages start to get embarrassing! The common denominator in our bad relationships was us. No one else to blame. Taking responsibility helped us manage the emotional baggage we both brought to this relationship. It took some time to recognize that the parts we played in our past relationships did not apply to this one. We realized we could use what we learned about our own patterns from past experiences to make this relationship an entirely different animal. In the past, there were always imbalances in power between ourselves and our significant others. Settling into dominant or submissive roles was not an option for us. Parenting or being parented by one's significant other is not what a mature relationship should look like. I take responsibility for myself, and Erica does the same. We do not play games or engage in power plays. When things go south, our goal is to resolve the conflict, not to win the fight.

WE ARE GENUINE PARTNERS.

Erica and I are complete, fully-functioning adults with or without each other. Neither of us needs or desires to be in charge of the other. We are partners in the truest sense of the word.

In a successful romantic relationship, you can not have it both ways. You can either be in a parent-child relationship or a partnership relationship. *Partnership* does not mean that you both take the helm simultaneously. It means that your process is democratic so that whoever takes the lead on a project consults with their partner before making big decisions.

As we go about our daily chores, we have a rule we employ that has saved us tons of grief, "You can do it. I can do it. But you can't ask me to do it and also tell me how to do it." For example, I fold towels one way, and Erica folds them another. If I want her to fold the towels, I cannot also make her fold them my way. If she wants me to wash the dishes, she cannot also tell me how I should wash the dishes.

Conversely, true partners appreciate the talents the other person brings to the table. I am a pretty effective writer but weak when it comes to design. *A Guide for Aging Heroes* is written mainly by me and edited by Erica. The reverse is true for the design of our website and social media. We love learning from each other and have opened each other to new worlds of knowledge and insight as a result.

WE OWN OUR SHIT.

A kid asked me once what it meant to be an adult. I said that when kids screw up, they blame others or make excuses. When grownups screw up, they take responsibility and try to do better next time. For Erica and me, when things go sideways, our first internal response is, "Is this my shit?"

Did I miscommunicate?

Did I misinterpret what was said?

Am I overreacting?

Am I in a bad mood?

Am I angry about something else and projecting it onto this situation?

How did I contribute to this conflict?

Am I hangry?

What can I do differently next time?

This sounds simple, but it takes a great deal of self-awareness. It is human nature to blame negative feelings on others. If I feel angry, then obviously, someone or something "made" me angry. Right? Likewise, if I feel frustrated, sad, or anxious.

In truth, your moods usually result from your neurochemistry and often have little to do with events outside of yourself. Incidents that are typically only slightly annoying to you can become huge issues when you are in a negative mood state. If you have negative feelings, own them, then take measures to prevent harm to your relationships.

WE PLAY BY THE RULES.

You may have noticed the same dramas playing out over and over again in your relationships. Your conflicts may have to do with financial matters, household responsibilities, jealousy, child-rearing differences, control issues, or any number of other relationship conflict themes. Whatever the problem, adhering to some basic rules can help you navigate the rough waters.

- No name-calling, blaming, or otherwise attacking the character of your partner. Ad Hominem attacks do nothing to resolve a conflict and can result in long-term hard feelings. You can't put the genie back in the bottle once you have said something hurtful.

- Do not try to resolve problems when you or your partner are upset. A primitive part of your brain is activated when you are upset and tends to short-circuit the reason and problem-solving centers. Both partners should agree to back off at the request of the other and resume when things cool down.

- Own your shit. Is this the same conflict you had with past partners or other people in your life? If so, this may be your shit! Again, feeling true and being true are often not the same thing. Feeling jealous doesn't mean you have something to be jealous about. Feeling angry doesn't mean your anger is justified. Feeling scared does not mean you are in danger. Trying to view the situation from the eyes of an imaginary third party can be a helpful strategy for recognizing your issues.

- Present possible solutions to the problem. "What can I do to resolve this?" or "This is what I would like for you to do to resolve this." Once you and your partner agree on a strategy, STICK TO IT.

- Respect what your partner says they want from you and

don't be skittish about asking exactly what that might be. Resolving the problem, NOT winning the conflict, should always be your ultimate goal.

NOTEBOOK ACTIVITY: SHARE THIS CHAPTER

If you are currently in a romantic relationship, go over this chapter with your partner. If you are not in a romantic relationship, share the chapter with a friend or family member who is. Write down what the experience of sharing the chapter was like. Successful romantic relationships require flexibility, communication, respect, love, and humility. The quality of your romantic relationships can determine the quality of a big part of your life. What are you doing right in your relationships? How could you improve?

DAY 22: ESTABLISH INTIMACY

"Fear is the great enemy of intimacy. Fear makes us run away from each other or cling to each other but does not create true intimacy."[cx]
~ Henri Nouwen

Erica and I are fortunate to share a dynamic and intimate relationship. We are physically intimate when we touch each other. We are intellectually intimate when we explore ideas together. We are aesthetically intimate when we appreciate things we find beautiful together. We are emotionally intimate when we experience our joys and sorrows together. Intimacy can die if it is not nurtured. We all have a friend we have allowed to go by the wayside because we didn't make the effort to keep the relationship intact.

Touch is a powerful aspect of human intimacy. We are wired for touch. While children are sometimes scolded for touching or picking up items in stores, we adults must admit that we engage in the same behavior. When I see something cool in a store, I want to pick it up. I used to live out in the country in Hollywood, South Carolina. I had a neighbor who had monkeys! I remember visiting the monkeys and sitting close to them. One of the monkeys came over and started grooming my hair. He would pick at my hair and then lick the tips of his fingers. After a while, the monkey stopped and leaned his back toward me. He was communicating that now it was my turn to groom him. I complied. Primates spend up to twenty percent of their day grooming each other.

I once met a group of gypsy hippies who traveled together from one music festival to the next. They were kind, free-spirited folks who operated well outside of the mainstream. I had a lot of fun playing music, singing, and dancing with them. One thing I noticed is that they were always touching each other. They did each other's hair, hugged, high-fived, and gave each other massages. I thought it was really sweet. Some physical touch relates to cultural norms. When people from Southern Europe, Russia, and the Middle East interact, they frequently touch each other. On the other hand, people in Great Britain and the US are generally much less likely to casually touch each other during conversations. Of course, these are generalizations and can never predict an individual's behavior from any culture.

Touch promotes trust, social bonding, and even generosity.[cxi] [cxii] It also soothes people who feel isolated or afraid. Touch can be a language of compassion.[cxiii] When a person pets a dog, positive endorphins, happy neurochemicals, are released in both the dog and the human! Unfortunately, creeps have created such litigious societies that folks feel reluctant to connect through touch. I hug, pat backs, scruff hair, and generally engage in a lot of physical touch with the people I know and love. However, with casual acquaintances and strangers, I ask permission. Not everyone is comfortable receiving physical contact from people they don't know well, and that's ok.

I am a pretty cerebral guy and stay stuck in my mind much of the time. When I lay my head on Erica's lap and she plays with my hair, it always brings me back to the present moment. Erica and I connect and reconnect constantly. We kiss, hug, and scratch each other's backs. We play with each other's ears. We touch each other's faces. We look deep into each other's eyes. We make love.

A stage of social development that usually happens during young adulthood (but can happen at any time in life) is called intimacy versus isolation.[cxiv] The successful outcome at this stage is intimacy. The term often implies a sexual relationship, but in this case, it doesn't necessarily mean that. For social development, intimacy simply means a relationship wherein you trust another person enough to allow yourself to be vulnerable, and they trust you in the same way. Success in this stage means that you have at least one person in your life with whom you feel safe to share your deepest fears and secrets. Established couples who disclose more about themselves "are more loving, more satisfied with their relationships, and more likely to stay together than couples who self-disclose less with each other."[cxv]

The humanist Sidney Jourard said, "It is through self-disclosure that an individual reveals to himself and to the other party just exactly who, what and where he is."[cxvi] I used to teach group therapy classes. One universal outcome was that, at some point, a group member would share that when she first entered the group, she assumed she was the only one with inner turmoil and everyone else in the group had their lives together. One error people make is comparing their internal experiences with what other people are showing on the outside. Everyone tends to "put on a good face" around unfamiliar people. In a successful therapy group, the participants gradually become comfortable sharing intimate aspects of their lives. Eventually, the truth that everyone is dealing with internal issues is revealed.

Failure to develop intimacy results in isolation. Isolation does not mean enjoying your own company or taking time out for yourself. Isolation is a fundamental lack of connection in the world. One manifestation of isolation can be depression. Depression occurs when isolated individuals turn negative feelings on themselves. Depression is but one possible result of isolation.

Intimacy grows from honest self-disclosure and avoidance of deception. Perfectionism can be a form of deception. It can serve as a duplicitous mask to hide self-doubt. If someone can make their external world look perfect, maybe they can fool people into thinking their inner world is also perfect. Likewise, bragging, lying, and being a know-it-all or a show-off are smokescreens to hide insecurities. Well-adjusted people are not afraid to acknowledge their weaknesses. Isolated people are self-absorbed and terrified of being found out. They may have lots of other folks in their lives, but others simply serve as objects to fulfill the isolated person's endless need for validation.

NOTEBOOK ACTIVITY: REACH OUT

Call or text a friend or family member you haven't heard from in a while. Write down your thoughts and feelings about the experience. I heard a story about researchers who wired a rat to biofeedback machines and then placed it in a bucket of water from which there was no escape. The rat swam around frantically, and its stress response was through the roof. All it took to bring the rat's bio readings back to normal was to put another rat in the bucket with it. Even in a no-win situation, social connection eases our suffering.

DAY 23: ENJOY SEX

"Don't be afraid. Don't be ashamed. Don't ever apologize for your sexuality. Just be you."[cxvii]
~ Sonya Deville

For Erica and me, sex is one way we connect. It serves as a means to express our love and to have fun together. As long as it is safe, legal, consensual, and for us, monogamous, anything goes.

An orgasm is the most powerful natural physical reward the body can give itself! As an added benefit, sex is also healthy for you.[cxviii] Sex improves your immune system, lowers your blood pressure, and decreases your risk of a heart attack. Sex can help with pain and stress management. Sex improves sleep and can even count as a part of your cardio workout! The rule of thumb for aging heroes is, "use it or lose it." The more sex you have (this includes masturbation), the more sex you can have. Your libido rises with your sexual frequency.

Sexual issues are pretty common. The most frequent sexual issue for men is erectile dysfunction or ED. Nearly all men will experience it at some time in their lives. Erectile dysfunction can be caused by psychological problems like anxiety or by physical conditions like injuries, low testosterone, or poor circulation. Since virility is tied closely to masculinity, ED can be emotionally devastating. Smoking, drinking, and obesity are all associated with increased erectile dysfunction. I have suffered from this issue, and it cut me to the core. Fortunately, we live in a time when ED can be treated. Oral drugs, penile injections, penile suppositories, vacuum erection devices, hormone therapy, and surgical implants are all options used to treat ED. Also, there are lots of things people can do sexually that don't require an erect penis.

For women, the most frequent problem is hypoactive sexual disorder. This just means low sex drive. As with ED in men, female hypoactive sexual disorder can have psychological or physical causes. Arthritis, circulatory problems, certain medications, and physical fatigue can harm the sex drive. Sex drive in men and women results from testosterone. Since women generally have less of it than men, it is understandable that low sex drive is a common issue. Hormones aside, guilt, shame, low self-esteem, body image issues, and negative past experiences are persistent culprits affecting female sex drive. Years ago, Erica was a victim of sexual assault. These events had a crushing impact on Erica's relationship with sex for many years.

As with men, sexual issues in women can be embarrassing. Emotional hang-ups are probably the biggest obstacles to a satisfying sex life, regardless of gender. If both partners are open, there are usually workarounds to most sexual difficulties. Because sex issues can be awkward, reluctance to seek treatment and poor communication with sex partners can be significant barriers to men and women successfully working through sexual problems.

Socially, sex is a taboo topic. This may be partly because sex is addressed as a moral issue in most world religions. The specifics of religious moral rules governing sexual behavior differ drastically across time and culture. Before agriculture, when prehistoric tribes were hunters and gatherers, there is evidence that people enjoyed equality and sexual freedom.[cxix] Males and females had sex partners of their choosing, and sex was not considered an aspect of morality. Sex may have been considered a bodily function like eating, breathing, and sleeping. Hunters and gatherers lived day-to-day on what they could find, so there was little accumulation of wealth. Therefore, there was no property to fight over or to "keep in the family." Tribes survived because everyone worked together for the benefit of everyone else. With no competition within tribes, tribe members were treated as equals.

With agriculture came ownership of land and livestock, permanent housing, and the desire to amass assets. When resources became limited, people had to compete for them. One theory is that as people competed for commodities, men grew in dominance simply because they were bigger and stronger.[cxx] New religions arose, reflecting these male-dominated societies. Religious morality provided rules, such as gender-based inheritance, that improved the opportunity to keep wealth within a family. Ultimately, women became just another commodity. They were properties to be held or traded. While things have improved considerably, the patriarchal attitude that men are more important than women still prevails today.

In many families, male children continue to be favored over female children. My paternal grandmother had numerous brothers and sisters. Her brothers were all put through college by their parents and received all of the inheritance. The girls in the family were expected to marry men who would provide for them.

The cliché that mothers blame their son's marital issues on the women they married, regardless of how badly said sons behaved, still rings true. Evil women corrupting otherwise good men is a theme that stretches across human history. The story of Samson and Delilah is an excellent example of this.

Sexual moral rules stemming from religion may have improved life by strengthening families, decreasing unwanted pregnancies, and slowing the spread of STDs. But they have also done much harm. Many religions inspire bigotry regarding sexual orientation and gender. Religious moral rules about sexuality typically benefit men at the expense of women. Sexual prowess continues to be a desirable trait for men but a scandalous one for women. In some cultures, women are still treated as the property of men. There are religious groups who place the blame for sexual assault on the women who were assaulted! Religious sexual rules favoring men have led to many women feeling guilt and shame about their sexuality. The frequency of sexual dysfunction in women is directly related to the level of gender inequality in a region.[cxxi] Higher degrees of religious influence in cultures and individuals are associated with more sexual guilt and shame.[cxxii] In other words, the more religious a person is, the more likely she is to suffer shame and guilt about her sexuality.

So, how is an aging hero supposed to manage? Aging heroes navigate sexuality as they do all of life's domains. They reject conformity for its own sake and go their own way. Communicate with your partner, experiment, see a doctor if you need to, and try new things. Leave no stone unturned. Have fun!

NOTEBOOK ACTIVITY: ENJOY SEX

Enjoy one sexual experience either with your partner or by yourself. Be creative, and maybe try something a little different. If the act or thoughts about the act cause any shame or guilt, use your CBT skills from Day 7 to override those irrational emotions. Sex can be one of life's greatest pleasures. It's important. Morally, apply your personal code of honor to sexual issues. Ask yourself the three questions: Is harm done? Is it fair? Am I being empathetic? Rather than living within the tiny box of how people are "supposed to be" sexually, find what works for you (and your partner if you have one) and appreciate the wonder that comes with being sexually free.

DAY 24: STAY CONNECTED

"The business of business is relationships; the business of life is human connection."[cxxiii]

~ Robin S. Sharma

The COVID-19 pandemic caused a less publicized epidemic, loneliness. Social distancing and social isolation were necessary to decrease the spread of the virus, but also may have caused some people to lose vital connections with other human beings. This may sound more like an inconvenience than a crisis, but the potential consequences of isolation can be deadly.

Believe it or not, 30 years of research have proven that *loneliness carries a similar risk for early death as smoking and high blood pressure!*[cxxiv] It is surprising that with this mother lode of evidence that more doctors are not prescribing increased social involvement to their patients. The health risks are equally dangerous whether someone is physically alone or merely *feels* lonely and disconnected despite having people around.

Social isolation affects adults and children alike. After World War II, the number of orphans in France had grown dramatically. At the same time, there was a shortage of caregivers and healthcare workers. The death rate for infants in institutions was staggering, sometimes 100%. Most of these children did not die from poor nutrition, physical illness, or abuse. They died from a condition called "failure to thrive," caused by social isolation. Children who did not perish in the orphanages were often physically stunted and had severe emotional problems. In recent studies, the growth rates of premature infants massaged for 15 minutes three times per day were 47% higher than children left alone in incubators.[cxxv] Children require more than food and shelter to survive. They need human contact. They need to be held. They need to be talked to and sung to.

Social contact is a vital component of health and wellness for children and adults. Our relationships ground us, define us, and give our lives meaning. The number of personal interactions we have in a day is directly related to our sense of happiness and well-being for that day.[cxxvi] Erica has historically preferred to live in town. She says the hustle and bustle of people going about their business gives her a greater sense of social connection. In the small town where she grew up, Erica knows everyone. She is guaranteed to run into friends and acquaintances when she walks the dogs.

Staying socially connected is easier if you are working or going to school. Outside of that, joining groups with similar interests to yours can be a lot of fun. There are groups for every hobby, from rock climbing to butterfly collecting. There are also church and community groups. But how do you stay connected when you can't get out of the house? Here are some lifelines:

Deepen your relationships. If you are fortunate enough to live with other people, strengthen those relationships. Talk about feelings. Express appreciation. Ask if the people in your life are ok.

Be self-aware. Life becomes very small in isolation. Little things become big things. Little annoyances become big annoyances. Tune in to how living in isolation relates to your own emotional experiences, and don't blame others when you have negative feelings.

Use technology. Reaching out to others by phone, video chat, email, or social media can be highly therapeutic. Sometimes a simple phone call can transform anxiety and depression into security and optimism.

Get creative. Use digital media to share art, music, and other creative projects with your friends and family. Two of our three adult children who live away from us are musicians. They have both done live video streams, and we were able to interact with them during the shows through messaging. Erica and our youngest child have some kind of digital conversation every day.

Join online groups. If you are not the joining type, maybe it is time to change that. Whatever interests you have, there are digital media groups that share them. I joined fitness, sailing, political, motorcycling, and humanitarian groups. It is wonderful to connect with like-minded folks.

NOTEBOOK ACTIVITY: BROADEN YOUR HORIZONS

Write down a few new ways to connect with others, then try one of them out. Use suggestions from this chapter or come up with some of your own. Social isolation can be devastating for some. We must be proactive when there are diminished natural opportunities for human interaction. By utilizing healthy strategies for connecting and reconnecting with others, we can counteract many of the hazards that accompany loneliness. Let's help each other get through difficult times. Reach out to people and ask them to reach out to you.

DAY 25: BE AN INDIVIDUAL

"Most people are other people. Their thoughts are someone else's
opinions, their lives a mimicry, their passions a quotation"
~ Oscar Wilde

As I shared in the preface, Erica and I had an ongoing discussion
about the term *cool* that eventually led to the concept of the Aging
Hero. We decided that there are no universals when it comes to cool.
Cool is subjective. As long as you are authentic, cool is what *you* are
passionate about. If upcycling well-worn sweaters is your passion,
then upcycling well-worn sweaters is cool. If dumpster diving is
your thing, then dumpster diving is cool.

On the other hand, uncool has a universal litmus: conformity.
Conformity, for its own sake, is uncool and unheroic. It springs
from fear of rejection. Rollo May said, "The opposite of courage in
our society is not cowardice; it is conformity."[cxxvii]

Where I grew up on the sea islands of South Carolina, there was
a prescribed look for men. *Real men* kept their hair short. If a guy
wanted to "look nice," he wore khaki pants, a knit shirt, and boat
shoes. The fashion was a billed trucker cap, jeans or camouflage, a t-
shirt, and boots on less formal occasions. You might have been
judged unmanly if you didn't follow the unwritten dress code. The
guys I grew up with were terrified of being considered unmanly.
Neither I nor any of my friends broke the dress code. To be
considered manly (check the irony here), a guy had to be too scared
to wear what he wanted. It turns out that we were cowards when it
came to individuality!

During a training run, Erica and I processed this idea of individuality in terms of *style*. I am not particularly tuned in on the style front, but I'm curious and open to learning. On the other hand, Erica has a good deal of experience and talent in this arena. Even as a young child, Erica excelled at expressing her sense of style. Over the years, she worked on and off as a fashion model and designer.

She describes her modeling years as disastrous to her self-esteem. While the public might view the life of a fashion model as glamorous, Erica says, for her, it was anything but. Models are often treated as inanimate objects or "glorified coat hangers." Photographers would be looking for specific features to fulfill their vision for a shoot. Disparagements of models were made in conversations between executives and photographers as if the models were not in the room. Often, the criticisms were about things a model had no control over. Erica was criticized for having too light skin on one shoot and too dark skin on another. "They might like my walk but not like the shape of my nose. Or, they liked the texture of my hair but didn't feel like people would be relatable. I was sometimes filtered out at a morning go-see for being too thin and filtered out that afternoon for being too heavy. The unhealthy discovery of sugar-free gum, caffeine, and laxatives as my sole intake for the day became a cycle that I battled for years."

Erica indicated that photographers often wanted models to fill ethnic roles. They wanted a Caucasian, a Latino, an African American, and an Asian model to cover ethnic bases. Consumers need to be able to identify and see themselves in the models used to market products. Erica is bi-racial, so she did not fit well into any of the ethnic boxes. Erica felt that modeling forced her to be inauthentic. "Being a model was like wearing a mask. I had to play roles, and they always made me feel like I wasn't being true to myself."

Erica says that while the terms are often used interchangeably, fashion and style are entirely different concepts. Fashion is whatever is popular at a given time, while style is a form of self-expression.

Yves Saint Laurent said, "Fashions fade. Style is eternal."[cxxviii] *Style* and *cool* seem to go hand in hand. Style may take courage to pull off as it can conflict with social norms. Fashion requires zero courage. Fashion is conformity for its own sake.

Think back to high school. Did you rebel against your parent's values? Was it a time of confusion for you? If so, you probably accomplished a critical stage of development, *identity formation*. If not, it is never too late! Successful identity formation is a prerequisite for aging heroes.

If you want concrete answers to questions about which is the best religion, political party, or sports team, ask a fifth grader. For a fifth-grader, the answers are clear-cut. The answers to these questions are whatever the fifth grader's parents say they are. Fifth graders tend to perfectly reflect their parents' values.

Along with many other physical changes, a lot of brain growth happens in adolescence. Suddenly, teens can think more abstractly and see gray areas where before, they only saw black and white. They recognize that their parents are not right about everything. And, if they are wrong about some things, maybe they are wrong about everything?! This can be a challenging time for parents and teenagers, but it is also necessary.

Healthy teens go through a stage of questioning their parents' values. Their next move is often a switch from copying their parents to copying their friends. Go to any high school, and you will see remarkable uniformity in how the students rebel. Clothing, hair, music, and even how they speak are affected by the need to fit in with their peers. Conformity for its own sake is one step many young people take on their path to *identity formation*. Identity formation is the process of becoming a distinct self, independent of friends and family. At some point along the way, well-adjusted teens will accept the parts of their parent's and friends' values that feel like a good fit and will reject the parts that don't. What emerges is a person with a unique identity. Alan Watts said, "When a man no longer confuses himself with the definition of himself that others have given him, he is at once universal and unique."[cxxix] Do you have the same religious and political affiliations as the people who raised you? If so, do you think that is a coincidence?

Unfortunately, not everyone makes it through the identity formation process. Some people wind up in *identity foreclosure*. They never question the values they grew up with and remain identity fifth-graders forever! Rather than actively exploring identity during adolescence, they just accepted whatever they were told. Foreclosed people do a lot of harm in the world. They tend to have high rates of conformity, bigotry, authoritarianism, and defensive narcissism.[cxxx] Authoritarianism means blind obedience to those you identify with as leaders. Defensive narcissism is a smug veneer of self-righteousness and a lack of empathy for people you see as different from you. Foreclosed people bulldoze through life with little awareness of the destruction they cause. Occasionally, however, time shines a light on unexamined lives. In old age, foreclosed folks are often full of regrets. This is tragic as it is sometimes too late to repair the damage.

People in identity foreclosure are governed by fear and conformity. Have you met grown-ups who carried into adulthood the high school obsession with having the right clothes, shoes, houses, and cars? They still desperately want to fit in, and they think keeping up with the Joneses is the way to do it. Competing for who has the best stuff is normal in adolescence, but when this juvenile behavior is carried into adult life, it is a recipe for misery all the way around. *Things* are a hollow substitute for character. Foreclosed people are incapable of genuine self-expression because they never formed a unique identity. Style and cool are not accessible to the foreclosed.

Expressing yourself may be challenging even if you have done the work to form a unique identity. We are all influenced by the people around us, and society does place limitations on self-expression. I worked as a college instructor, and Erica as a hospital administrator. If we wanted to express ourselves by showing up for work in bathing suits, our employers might suggest we seek therapy! Also, for better or worse, it is human nature to make snap judgments about people we don't know based only on their appearance. You will be judged by your appearance. When I look and dress like a biker, I get very different responses from people than when I look and dress like a college professor. I am the same person, but people judge me differently. As a true aging hero, my internal response to such judgments is, "So what?" *What's most important when addressing individuality is how you see yourself.*

NOTEBOOK ACTIVITY: EXPRESS YOURSELF

Use style to express your individuality in a way you never have before. Make it simple but personal. Find what feels right to you and enjoy style as an opportunity to communicate who you are to the world. The process can be very freeing. Write down how the change made you feel. Style is an area of life that I never explored until Erica and I got together. It is a lot of fun to stretch a bit beyond my *real man* attire. Erica's style is often an expression of how she feels on a particular day.

DAY 26: COLLABORATE

"When you need to innovate, you need collaboration."
~ Marissa Mayer

Collaboration and holism go hand in hand. Collaboration is an intelligent way to operate because the whole is always greater than the sum of its parts. I consider myself a pretty smart fellow with a lot of life experience. But I am only one guy with one perspective and one life to draw from. I have found that 100% of the time, a room full of first-year college students can develop more novel solutions to a social problem than I can ever come up with on my own. I am fascinated by ideas and love it when others spark a new perspective on an issue. It is humbling at my age to continue to learn from 18-year-olds. Holism: a room full of students with their teacher is smarter than the teacher or any individual student.

I heard that when one of the Beatles brought a new song to the rest of the band, the song was transformed into something completely different. Separately, the Beatles were all talented musicians, but together they were the Beatles! Holism: the talent of the Beatles is greater than any one of the band's members.

Around the turn of the century, there was a social scientist named Sir Francis Galton. Sir Francis discovered what has come to be called *the wisdom of the crowd*. As the story goes, Galton was at a county fair, and a game was played where villagers tried to guess the weight of an ox. Sir Francis collected the guesses from close to 800 people. What he found when he processed this data was incredible.

None of the guessers, not even livestock breeders, came close to the ox's actual weight, 1,197 pounds. Get this. When Galton averaged all of the guesses together, the result was 1,196 pounds! Holism: the crowd was smarter than any person in that crowd.

Erica and I compete in dragon boat races. The boats look like long canoes with ten bench seats and a carved dragon head on the prow. Twenty paddlers sit two abreast with a drummer in the bow of the boat to beat time and a helmsman steering in the stern. The races are 250m, 500m, or 2000m sprints. Getting 20 people to work together is more complicated than you might think. In the excitement of a race, inexperienced crew members will start stroking as fast as they can and lose track of what the rest of the team is doing. This is the kiss of death. When a dragon boat crew perfectly synchronizes their movements and pulls hard together, they can reach speeds of up to 15 kph. That is faster than our sailboat in a heavy wind! A physically weak crew can win a race against a physically strong crew if the weak crew works together and the strong crew does not. Holism: a physically weak crew working together is faster than a physically strong crew working independently.

Bosses who make changes without getting input from the people doing the work are screw-ups, regardless of the size of the business. Wise leaders respect the expertise of others and get as much feedback as possible from knowledgeable people before making big decisions. In your associations, remember to appreciate what others bring to the table. It is foolish and arrogant to do otherwise. People who have to have everything their way are emotionally immature. That kind of egocentrism should be reserved for toddlers. All relations require collaboration and compromise. This is true for employers, co-workers, romantic partners, families, and friends.

You don't need 800 people for the wisdom of the crowd to work. Erica and I make for a damned small crowd, but holism proves true every time we collaborate on a project. We are both creative people but creative in very different ways. I am creative with words, and Erica is with images. She has given me an appreciation for visual aesthetics. Something that I was never aware of before we connected. When watching movies, we both appreciate the total package presented in a film. But, I attend mainly to the dialogue, the story, and the acting, while Erica is more interested in the sets, costumes, music, and camera techniques. When we work together, we create something neither of us could have formed on our own. Holism.

Collaborative cooperation might take a little practice, or it might take a lot. Some people are better at it than others. Erica and I are both very flexible, so working together usually goes smoothly. We use the metaphor of removing our personal hats and putting on our business hats whenever we are working on a professional project together. Ideas shared when we are in our business hats are strictly business and never personal. The more rigid individual collaborators are, the more frustrating the process can become. On the rare occasion when I "know I'm right" on one side of an issue and Erica "knows she's right" on the other side of the issue, we run into trouble. When that happens, we must look at ourselves and check our egos. We must reevaluate the merits of our own positions and make a concerted effort to approach the opposing position with fresh eyes. We had several stalemates in the creation of this book. Ultimately, our process worked, and one or the other of us yielded or compromised as we saw fit. Often, folks will double down on an inferior idea purely based on it being their idea. Doubling down is generally a red flag for immaturity. Erica and I switch gears and take time to reflect rather than doubling down on an idea about which we disagree. This is a product of mutual respect for one another.

NOTEBOOK ACTIVITY: HOLISM

The gifts of successful collaboration are meaningful shared social experiences and successful outcomes. Write down times when "the whole is greater than the sum of its parts" was proven true in your life. What opportunities do you have to collaborate with others? Are you a good partner when it comes to collaboration?

BEING A PHYSICAL HERO

"When it comes to eating right and exercising, there is no 'I'll start tomorrow.' Tomorrow is disease."[cxxxi]
~ V.L. Allinear

At first blush, the mind and the body appear to be separate entities. They are not. In simple terms, the mind is what the brain does, and the brain is part of your physical body. Shut off the brain, and the mind ceases to exist. Stroke victims and people with brain damage are evidence enough that the mind is a product of the brain. As impressive as it is, the brain is just a physical organ like your liver, lungs, and kidneys. Physical health creates brain health, and brain health improves the mind's functioning.

Your body and brain are your instruments for experiencing life. They do not need to be sleek or fancy but should be well-tuned and reliable. The more efficient your physical machine is, the wider your range of possible activities becomes. People have different levels of interest in physical adventures. Erica and I are crazy about them, so we must stay in relatively good condition. If your interests gravitate toward less strenuous activities, maintain a level of fitness that will ensure you can enjoy those activities for years to come. If walking the dog around the neighborhood gives you great pleasure, you don't need to be in shape to run a marathon. You do, however, need to train your strength, balance, endurance, and flexibility sufficiently to continue to walk that pup far into the future.

DAY 27: IMPERFECT VESSELS

"Start where you are. Use what you have. Do what you can."
~ Arthur Ashe

Physical health is a bedrock for wellness. You may think that exceptionally fit people are qualitatively different from you. Maybe they are younger, have more time, better genes, or fewer physical maladies than you. In truth, superior fitness is accessible to most of us. We all get the same 24-hour day. Genes are rarely a legitimate barrier to attaining phenomenal physical conditioning. And as for health problems, you don't become an aging hero without taking some hard knocks. Erica and I are not exceptions. Here are a few of our issues.

Rusty:
COPD
Deformed vertebrae from a motorcycle accident
Arthritis
A missing tendon in one calf from an old injury
Major depression

Erica:
Hemiplegic migraines
Chronic injuries in both hips and knees
Chronic injury to left foot
Eating disorder

TIME IS NOT AN OBSTACLE!

Urige Buta, the Norwegian champion marathon runner, also worked as a janitor 10 hours a day to provide for his wife and young child. You can't possibly appreciate Mr. Buta's fantastic feat if you haven't trained for a marathon. Marathon training requires running for hours most days, followed by periods of extreme exhaustion. Working 10-hour shifts while training for marathons is incomprehensible!

Before achieving fame and fortune as an actress and the biggest name in mixed martial arts, Rhonda Rousey worked three bartending jobs at once while also training and competing in the MMA. Rhonda Rousey not only achieved success in a sport formerly dominated by men but also advanced the sport more than any athlete, male or female!

A recent study found that busyness improves the brain.[cxxxii] Busy people were found to have "better processing speed, working memory, episodic memory, reasoning, and crystallized intelligence" than their less engaged counterparts. In the same way that working the body improves physical performance, working the brain enhances its abilities.

AGE IS NOT AN OBSTACLE!

Tamae Watanabe was 63 when she broke the world record as the oldest woman to climb Mount Everest. At 73, she scaled Everest again and broke her own record! Climbing Mt Everest represents a capstone achievement for most climbers regardless of age. For Tamae Watanabe to do it twice and break the age barrier both times is beyond incredible!

Sixty-eight-year-old Cathy Skott rode her recumbent bicycle from Miami to Maine with Myron, her husband of forty years. They averaged biking 50 to 60 miles per day during the trips. In less than two months, she completed the 2,300-mile trek!

Ernestine Shepherd was overweight and suffered from depression, panic attacks, high blood pressure, and GERD. She and her sister started working out when Ernestine was age 56. She said, "Instead of lamenting about our bodies, we decided to make a change, get into shape and become the best version of ourselves."[cxxxiii] Through exercise and diet, Ernestine was able to stop taking medications for her health problems. She became a competitive bodybuilder and competed until age 80. After winning many titles, she retired as the world's oldest female bodybuilder. Now in her mid-eighties, Ernestine continues strength training for 45 minutes to an hour 4 times per week, and she runs 10 miles every morning!

Many of the conditions considered to be caused by aging are related in large part to disuse. Exercise improves every aspect of heart and circulatory function, increases bone density, improves muscle mass and strength, improves metabolism, decreases body fat, regulates insulin and blood sugar levels, decreases bad cholesterol, increases good cholesterol, improves sleep quality, and decreases depression and memory lapses. Exercise reduces the risks of stroke, heart disease, and even cancer!

HEALTH ISSUES ARE NOT OBSTACLES!

The swimmer, Eric Shanteau, won an Olympic medal for breaststroke in 2004. He then competed in the 2008 Olympics two weeks after being diagnosed with testicular cancer. Eric had chemotherapy after competing, was cancer-free before the year was out, and won Olympic gold in the swimming relay in 2012.

Despite pain and fatigue caused by the autoimmune disease, lupus, Shannon Box is a three-time Olympic gold medal winner and a highly decorated player in US women's soccer. After suffering for years, Shannon went public about her condition before the 2012 Olympics, where she helped her team win the gold. She continued to compete until 2015 and retired at age 35 after her team won the World Cup.

With chronic Crohn's disease, Carrie Johnson competed in the 2004 and 2008 Olympics in the 200 and 500-meter kayak events. She then won gold in the 2012 Pan American Games. She was the first person to qualify for her event for the 2012 Olympic Team. Carrie is quoted as saying, "Falling in life is unavoidable. Staying down is optional."[cxxxiv]

Scott Hamilton was adopted at the age of six weeks. He contracted a mysterious disease at two years old that stunted his growth. The condition was corrected with diet and exercise and was later found to be caused by a congenital brain tumor. Scott went on to win four US Championships, four World Championships, and an Olympic gold medal in figure skating. Hamilton says, "the only disability is a bad attitude."[cxxxv]

In 2003, Dana Vollmer had surgery to correct a heart condition called supraventricular tachycardia. She later won an Olympic gold medal for swimming as well as a gold medal in the World Aquatics Championships. At the time of this writing, she holds the world record for the 110-meter butterfly. Volmer's motto? "It's what you do with the rough patches that will define what kind of athlete you'll become."[cxxxvi]

Wilma Rudolph, who became known as "the fastest woman in the world" in the 1960s, required physical therapy due to childhood polio. Wilma was the first woman to win three Olympic gold medals in the same Games.

After having a stroke at age 36, Russell Winwood heeded the wake-up call and immersed himself in physical fitness. For about eight years, he competed as a triathlete and marathon runner. When he noticed that he was often short of breath, he went in for a medical checkup and was diagnosed with Stage 4 COPD. Stage 4 means that lung function is below 30 percent. Six months after this crushing diagnosis, Russell competed in his first full ironman race! As a fellow sufferer of COPD, Russell Winward is one of my heroes!

According to the Mayo Clinic, exercise can reduce heart disease, diabetes, asthma, back problems, and arthritis symptoms. Exercise also improves mental health. The National Center for Biotechnology Information indicates that anxiety, depression, and negative mood can all be reduced through exercise by improving self-esteem and cognitive functioning.

Regardless of your age, your job, and your current level of fitness, you have the potential to make dramatic improvements! I have realized that my mind is the only genuine barrier to my success.

NOTEBOOK ACTIVITY: WHO'S YOUR HERO?

Write down someone you admire from your life or the media who has overcome age, health problems, or time constraints to do something great. If that person can surmount obstacles, so can you! Have you ever used time, health, or age as excuses to keep you from doing something you really wanted to do? I shared with Erica that I had no idea what I was doing the first time I stood up in front of a college class to teach. I had no training as a teacher, but I did have a strategy. I role-played my favorite high school teacher, Carl Tutt. I used Mr. Tutt's vocal inflections, dramatic pauses, and habit of walking around the room as he lectured. These behaviors quickly became integrated into my own unique teaching style. Erica, in turn, used the same strategy to overcome performance anxiety at work. She was required to make presentations and actually role-played me! I'm paying it forward, Mr. Tutt! Choose your own heroes and channel them to establish the habits you desire.

DAY 28: GET IN SHAPE

"The best training program in the world is worthless without the will to execute it properly, consistently, and with intensity."[cxxxvii]
~ John Romaniello

There is no fountain of youth, but regular exercise and a healthy diet are pretty damn close. I was playing a music gig on the second floor of a restaurant a few years ago and recognized Sam, an elderly gentleman I knew from the gym. Sam was approaching 80 years old and hardly ever missed a workout. He is a very tall man, and his claim to fame was that he could still kick the top of a door frame. Sam was at the restaurant with a group of peers to celebrate a birthday. His friends were in the same age group, but they all seemed much older than him. Sam ran down to the first floor six times to help various friends climb the stairs and get to their table. I'm sure that if you asked Sam about a fountain of youth, he would point you to the gym.

Part of the Aging Heroes lifestyle is investing in experiences rather than possessions. The types of exploits Erica and I enjoy tend to involve physical activity. The more fit we are, the more able we are to engage in adventurous pursuits. I have always wanted to learn to surf. At 59, I finally made it happen. Well, Erica made it happen, as usual. We took a trip to Panama, and surfing lessons were part of the adventure. The trip also included hiking, swimming, snorkeling, and lots of walking. Without maintaining a certain level of fitness, many of the things we love to do will become less and less available to us as we age.

Together, Erica and I have over 40 years of serious workout experience. Erica is a runner who has participated in 100s of races. She competed in The Chicago and Mount Kilimanjaro Marathons. Working out has been a passion of mine since I was in my 30s. My physical transformation was dramatic when I started getting serious about training. At one point, I had a gym owner ask to use photos of me for marketing her health club.

Aging Heroes' physical training recommendations are not necessarily for bodybuilders and marathon runners. They are a set of guidelines for everyone. They will ensure that you meet the activity levels needed to improve and maintain your health and physical well-being. In all areas of life, aging heroes make their own way. Fitness is no exception. Design a unique workout routine for your specific needs. Per our guidelines, your physical training should require no more than a commitment of 200 minutes per week. That averages out to slightly less than 30 minutes per day. Before beginning any physical conditioning program, you should check in and get approval from your doctor.

A comprehensive fitness program should include five components:[cxxxviii]

Aerobic (Cardio)
Anaerobic (Strength)
Flexibility (Stretching)
Balance
Core Training

AEROBICS

Aerobic exercise is essential to long-term cardiovascular health. Regular aerobic work improves the functioning of your lungs, your heart, and your circulatory system. It also enhances the quality of your sleep and your mental health. As a guy with chronic lung disease, I can tell you that aerobic exercise has impacted my quality of life more than any medications I take for my condition.

The US Department of Health and Human Services recommends at least 150 minutes (about 20 minutes per day) of moderate aerobic activity or 75 minutes (about 10 minutes per day) of vigorous aerobic exercise per week. Any activity that gets your heart rate up for at least 10 minutes counts. Mix and match. Find activities that are meaningful and fun.

Here are some examples of moderate aerobic activities:

- Brisk walking
- Gardening
- Heavy cleaning
- Lawn mowing (push)
- Bicycling with light effort
- Doubles tennis
- Dancing
- Rollerblading
- Recreational swimming
- Sweeping, mopping, vacuuming

Here are examples of vigorous aerobic activities:

- Jogging or running
- Swimming laps
- Bicycling fast or on hills
- Singles tennis
- Basketball, football, rugby, soccer, hockey, racketball
- Gymnastics
- Martial arts
- Shoveling
- Jumping rope

Erica is the cardio expert in our family. She spent a big chunk of her life as a distance-running zealot. She has run the gamut of running-related injuries herself and has a long list of race training dos and don'ts. I have been a gym rat for a long time, but the fueling, hill work, running gear, training frequencies, rest periods, and diet required for distance running are a new world of knowledge for me. Erica trained me for several races. It was fun to work out together and learn the ropes of racing.

STRENGTH TRAINING

Don't be intimidated by strength training. You won't turn into Arnold Schwarzenegger. The time required for strength training is minimal, you will notice results very quickly, and the benefits to your long-term health can not be overstated. Strength training is necessary for anyone middle-aged or older. The average adult over 30 loses 3% to 5% of muscle mass every decade.[cxxxix] Less muscle mass means more weakness and less ability to get around. This increases your likelihood of falling and breaking bones. Strength training preserves muscle, increases bone density, and improves balance and coordination. It can also help you manage chronic conditions like arthritis, obesity, back problems, diabetes, and even mental illness.[cxl]

Traditionally, people who wanted to trim down were advised to add more cardio to their routines. Indeed, people who do more than 150 minutes of cardio per week have the best outcomes for weight loss. However, weight training increases muscle mass while burning fat. Muscle weighs more than fat, so the changes resulting from strength training may not always appear on the scales. Recent studies show that a combination of cardio and strength training is best for improving body composition and long-term weight control.[cxli] Cardio work tends to burn more calories per minute than strength training. However, the calorie-burning is also finished when the cardio workout is finished. With strength training, you burn fewer calories per minute during the workout, but you continue to burn calories for up to 48 hours after the activity is finished as your body recuperates. Also, strength training increases muscle mass, increasing resting metabolism, the calories you burn when doing nothing.

In strength training, you must work on each major muscle group at least once weekly. You can do a full-body workout that targets everything in one workout or split up the muscle groups and work them over several sessions.[cxlii] There are different ways to divide the muscle groups, but here is how I do it:

- Back
- Chest
- Shoulders
- Core
- Legs

I like to divide the muscle groups over several workouts. If I am doing two strength training workouts per week, I work the chest, shoulders, and core in one workout, then the legs, core, and back in the next workout. If I am doing strength training four times per week, I do chest and core one day, back one day, shoulders one day, and legs and core one day. Never work the same muscle group two days in a row. Rest each muscle group for at least one day between workouts.

Aging heroes need functional strength. Exercises that build functional strength simulate natural movements you would do in everyday life. Such compound movements hit several muscles at one time. For instance, when you do a bench press or pushup to build your chest, you use natural pushing movements that work your chest muscles and your triceps and deltoids. When you do bent-over rows to strengthen your back, you use natural pulling movements that hit your back muscles and your biceps and core. When you do squats and calf raises with weights or resistance bands, you are using natural, compound movements to work the muscles in your legs and your back, shoulders, and arms.

There are many strength training options available. Some people like to train with traditional barbells and dumbbells. I love dumbbells because they work the large muscles that give me strength and power and the small muscles used for coordination. Other folks prefer body-weight exercises like pushups, situps, pull-ups, and knee bends. Zac McGowen, who played the pirate, Captain Charles Vane, in the television series *Black Sails,* got into incredible shape using only bodyweight exercises.[cxliii] He didn't want to use equipment that was unavailable to people in the 1700s. Machines are another strength training option. Many gyms have weight machines you can use to train all of the major muscle groups. I have friends who are really into resistance bands. Resistance bands are lightweight, inexpensive, and can be used anywhere. You can buy rubber resistance tubes for less than fifty bucks and create an effective full-body workout.

Strength training workouts are measured in *reps* and *sets*. Reps are repetitions of a complete exercise movement. So, one pushup is one rep, and ten pushups are ten reps. A set is when you do several reps in a row. If you do ten reps of pushups, then rest and do another ten pushups, you have completed two sets of pushups. A good rule of thumb is to choose a resistance that allows you to complete about 12 reps. If you plan to do multiple sets of each exercise, rest for about one minute between sets. Starting out, 5 to 12 sets per strength training workout is plenty.[cxliv]

I like doing a 20-20-20 workout. Twenty minutes of strength training, 20 minutes of cardio, and 20 minutes of yoga stretching.

Doing this three or four times per week makes me feel at my best physically. I had to back my strength training down to once a week during marathon training. The time required for marathon training is insane. When you are not running, you are recovering from running.

STRETCHING

Flexibility is an often neglected aspect of fitness. When I was younger, if I was in a time crunch, stretching was the first thing I cut from my workout. As an older and wiser man, I give yoga the same attention as cardio and strength training. Stretching improves flexibility, helps circulate lymph through your body (which removes harmful waste and increases disease resistance), decreases muscle tension, and improves posture. It also reduces arterial stiffness, diastolic blood pressure, and heart rate.[cxlv] Stretching exercises should be done at least twice a week for at least 10 minutes. You should feel the stretch for each static stretching position but never to the point of it being painful.

Range of motion is how far you can stretch a part of your body.[cxlvi] It is the full movement potential of a joint. As children, we constantly used the full range of motion for all of our joints when we played outside. Games like tag, climbing on the monkey bars, sports, and tumbling in the grass stretched our ranges of motion regularly. For many of us, the movements we make in everyday life become more and more restricted as we grow older. Yoga stretches can help us maintain youthful ranges of motion.

There are two types of stretching. The first is static stretching, which is what most people think of when the topic of stretching comes up. Static stretches are poses held for a while to stretch specific muscles. For years, athletes were advised to do static stretches before an activity to decrease the risk of injuries. Later research showed that, in the short run, static stretches could reduce muscle power and increase an athlete's chance of injury if the athlete does them just before intense activities.[cxlvii] In the long run, static stretching improves athletic performance when done regularly. Static stretches should be used as a cool-down after your workout or as a separate, independent workout.

The second type of stretching is called dynamic stretching. Dynamic stretches involve actively moving joints through their full ranges of motion. Dynamic stretches help lubricate joints and warm muscles and tendons before strenuous activities. For instance, I do dynamic stretches by windmilling my arms in big circles before doing weight training to work my shoulders. Shadowboxing and calisthenics are also good examples of dynamic stretching.

I do yoga stretching at the end of every workout after my muscles have warmed up. Yoga is a great opportunity for me to practice mindfulness. I live in my body, but I tend to pay very little attention to my bodily sensations unless I get injured. Yoga tunes me into my breath and my body. I find yoga enjoyable on many levels. It helps me bring my mind into the present and quiet my thoughts, and many yoga positions just plain feel good. I have spent a lifetime tensing and contracting my muscles. It feels like a kindness to myself to stretch those muscles and give them some much-needed pull in the other direction.

You are in the game if you include the five components of cardio, strength, core, stability, and flexibility in your workout plan. Start where you are. If you are limited by health or mobility issues, design a routine that includes modifications to accommodate your specific needs. If standard aerobics is prohibited by arthritis, try water aerobics. If getting down on the floor for yoga is not possible, try chair yoga. Don't allow your perceived limitations to keep you from a well-rounded workout. As I have grown older, I have consistently modified which activities I choose for my workouts.

Break the cliche that portrays aging as a slow decline into decrepitude. Exercise will enable you to do the activities you love deep into old age. A body in motion tends to stay in motion, and a body at rest tends to remain at rest. Get moving! Name an outdoor adventure, and I'll show you 80 and 90-year-olds who are involved in it. Mountain climbing? Check out Enzo Appiano scaling the Alps at 90. Snowboarding? Ann Peacock was hitting the slopes in Colorado at 82. Hockey? Bill Parsley was still competing at 85! The profound improvements to your quality of life that will result from committing a little time to a well-rounded fitness routine cannot be overstated. Including cardio, strength training, and stretching into your weekly routine will cultivate power, confidence, health, mental abilities, and emotional stability. There is no downside!

NOTEBOOK ACTIVITY: YOUR FITNESS PLAN

This one might take a little time. Create a workout schedule that includes at least 200 minutes per week and covers strength training, cardio work, stretching, flexibility, balance, and core work. Balance and core work are included in strength training. The plan can be as involved or as simple as you like. There are many excellent apps to assist you if you are into collecting fitness data and tracking your workouts. We use Garmin Connect for cardio tracking, Jetfit for gym workouts, and Fitstar Stretching for flexibility. Once you establish your plan, stick to it. Don't make working out something you contemplate. Make it something you do automatically. Make it part of your lifestyle.

DAY 29: EAT WELL

"Healthy does NOT mean starving yourself EVER. Healthy means eating the right food in the right amount".
~ Karen Salmansohn

For Erica and me, maintaining a healthy diet is the most challenging aspect of wellness. Every day, everyone cycles through a wide range of physical and emotional states. We move through sleepy, angry, happy, sore, alert, scatterbrained, strong, tired, energetic, weak, sad, bored, overwhelmed, and on and on. Some of these states are conducive to making good life choices, others to making poor ones. Sticking to a workout plan is much easier than sticking to a diet. If I only have to choose to work out one time per day, a few times per week, and I am highly motivated, there is a pretty good likelihood that I will hit a state that leads to me making that choice. However, eating right requires making smart decisions regardless of my physical and mental state, 24/7. I have to override thousands of years of evolution. A pretty tall order!

Human beings evolved to survive in the natural environment. Food is never guaranteed in nature, so primitive people who ate heavy and stored fat when food was available tended to survive and stay in the gene pool. Fast forward to the modern age when many people have access to as much food as they desire, and you have a recipe for disaster. To make matters worse, food is integral to our social interactions. Every holiday is celebrated with eating and drinking. Also, we are inundated through the media with tempting ads for delicious food and drink. Evolutionary hardwiring moves modern humans to eat as much as possible and store the excess calories as fat.

Our research on diet revealed nothing new. Eat reasonable quantities of lean meats, whole grains, and lots of fresh fruits and vegetables. Avoid processed foods, sugar, hydrogenated oils, and fatty meats and dairy. All fad diets, including keto, low fat, fasting, and calorie restriction, can generate temporary weight loss. None have been shown to work over the long haul. So what is an aging hero to do?

Like most health-conscious people, Erica and I can easily differentiate between the foods that are good for us and those that aren't. Our diet issues didn't stem from a lack of knowledge, willpower, or commitment but from an unhealthy relationship with food. We ate out too much, and we self-stimulated by eating when we were over-tired, bored, or stressed.

To change our relationship with food, we began to practice mindful eating. We realized that we typically consumed meals with very little awareness. The food moved from table to stomach like a ghost. The experience of enjoying our food was lost because we were distracted by the television or a conversation or simply wanted to finish so we could move on to whatever was next on our agenda. There is a joke about a dog that ate its food so quickly that, when it finished, the dog looked around and growled because it assumed another dog had stolen it. Erica and I realized that we were missing out on one of life's sweetest pleasures by eating without conscious awareness.

Food scarcity remains an issue for many. I have had students who grew up in households without enough food to go around. For those of us with abundant access to food, eating should be a sacred act undertaken with deep appreciation. The privilege of consuming a nice meal deserves, at the very least, awareness of the process. Eating is not just a bodily function. It is an opportunity to experience something extraordinary that is denied to many.

A mindful approach to food should start with planning your meal. Enjoy mindfully selecting the items you will prepare. Consider that all food ultimately comes from the earth. Fruits, vegetables, nuts, and grains all grew up through the soil, drawing nutrients from the ground. Most of the meat people eat comes from vegetarian animals.

There is a horrible chicken processing plant in our town. Some days the stench carries for miles. The chickens are grown and butchered with no humanitarian regard. For us, part of mindful eating means choosing sources for our food that minimize the suffering of animals and use sustainable farming practices.

Preparing a meal mindfully can be an expansive experience. I once knew a young man who was a genius at origami. I asked him his secret as my attempts at origami always looked like a big mess. He said, "Do it like it is something important." I loved that advice. Prepare your meal as if what you are doing is important. Admire the colors, textures, and fragrances. Taste as you go and season accordingly. Enjoy the changes in temperature as steam rises from pots and pans. Remember that cooking for others is an act of love. Mindfully clean up behind yourself as you work.

When the food is ready, arrange it on plates in a visually pleasing way. Find a place to eat that is comfortable and free from distractions. Communicate your intention to experience the meal fully, with a humble sense of gratitude. Inhale the scents. Take in the visual aesthetics. Notice the weight of the plates and utensils as you handle them. Truly taste each bite and note what a wonderful thing it is to chew and swallow. Allow yourself to feel satisfied that you have done your body a kindness.

By shifting our attitudes about food, we can enjoy eating and never mindlessly gorge. The comedian Louis C.K. said, "I don't stop eating when I'm full. The meal isn't over when I'm full. I stop eating when I hate myself."[cxlviii] My grandmother used to end every meal by saying, "Well, I did it again. I feel like I'm going to burst!" Eating mindfully is a practice that naturally keeps you from overeating.

NOTEBOOK ACTIVITY: CLEANING UP AND TUNING IN

Go through your kitchen and remove unhealthy items. Get rid of unhealthy snacks, sodas, fatty meats and dairy, heavily processed foods, and non-whole grain flours, pastas, and baked goods. Keep only healthy cooking oils like canola and olive oil. There are also apps for menu planning.

Practice mindful eating for at least one meal per day. Record your experiences in your notebook.

DAY 30: GET HEALTHY SLEEP

"Each night, when I go to sleep, I die. And the next morning, when I wake up, I am reborn."[cxlix]
~Mahatma Gandhi

Sleep deprivation is one of the unfortunate side effects of making an ocean passage with a small crew. Because one sailor must always be on watch, a crew of two or three must stagger their sleep schedules. This can result in social stress, poor judgment calls, and increased careless errors. The same is true for understaffed Navy vessels. In 2017, there was a senate hearing regarding deadly accidents resulting from sleep-deprived sailors doing 100-hour workweeks while deployed overseas.[cl]

While you may not be crewing an ocean voyage, sleep disturbance can affect your quality of life, health, and daily functioning. Sleep deprivation may result in emotional instability, poor memory and concentration, compromised immunity, low sex drive, weight gain, high blood pressure, increased risk for diabetes, and even poor balance.[cli] Chronic sleep issues relate to increased mortality. Good sleep enhances problem-solving and insight. Signs that you are having sleep issues include yawning a lot, sleepiness during the day, low energy, and grouchiness.

So how much is the right amount for you? Well, the answer changes as you age.[clii] Young children can need over twice as much sleep as adults. For aging heroes, a proper night's sleep means from seven to nine hours per night. Quality of sleep is another factor to consider. If you wake up frequently during the night or have a sleep disorder like sleep apnea, where you snore and periodically gasp for breath while sleeping, you may still be sleep deprived even if you get enough hours in. If you think you may suffer from a sleep disorder, it is wise to consult with your doctor. Sleep clinics help diagnose and recommend treatments for various sleep disorders.

Humans evolved to sleep when it is dark and wake when it is light. I lived on James Island in 1989 when Hurricane Hugo struck. The experience was surreal. I had always assumed that radio and television broadcasts would instruct people on what to do when a catastrophic event occurred. There were none. The radio and television towers were destroyed. I assumed firefighters and law enforcement would be out in force helping out people in trouble. They eventually mobilized, but James Island looked like a ghost town right after the storm. I assume emergency personnel were taking care of their own families. The roads were all blocked by fallen trees, so transportation on the island was limited to foot traffic. Everyday life stressors like going to our jobs, buying groceries, and paying our bills were put on hold.

The days after the storm was like traveling back in time a couple of hundred years. Our daylight hours were spent sawing trees and removing debris. We ate huge meals cooked on barbeque grills and shared with others in the neighborhood as we needed to eat the food in our freezers before it spoiled. When the sun set, everyone went to bed. When the sun rose, we awoke, ate breakfast, and returned to working on tree removal again. I felt wonderful! I had never experienced such a sense of healthy balance. I think reverting to the sleep pattern of my distant ancestors recalibrated my psyche.

Part of understanding holism is recognizing that the macro reflects the micro and vice versa. In the macro, each life ends in death. In the micro, each day ends in sleep. This is the natural cycle and quite an elegant system. The same sense of wholeness and satisfaction that a person experiences at the end of a life well-lived can be experienced by each of us at the end of a day well-lived.

In dragon boating, we advise our crewmates with the phrase, "Leave it on the water!" Meaning pouring on every drop of strength and energy during a race so that you have nothing left after crossing the finish line. Each day, Erica and I try to "leave it on the water" by making our wake time count. We count a day spent sticking to our plans and living according to our personal philosophies and moral codes as a day well-lived.

Here are some tips for improving your sleep hygiene:

- Erica considers sleep from a design perspective. A tidy bedroom with crisp, clean sheets gives her a sense of comfort and stability.
- We also use guided imagery and relaxing music at bedtime.
- Stick to a sleep schedule. Go to sleep at the same time every night and have a fixed wake-up time. Make a nightly routine that prepares you for sleep.
- Make sleep a priority. Erica and I used to watch television in bed. She tended to doze off at the same time every night, but if I were not conscientious, I would become engrossed in a program and stay up too late.
- A good rule of thumb is to disengage from electronic devices a half hour to an hour before you plan to go to sleep. Tinkering on your phone or tablet can stimulate you and delay sleepiness.
- Some people are very noise sensitive and benefit from wearing earplugs when they sleep.
- Avoid caffeine in the afternoons and evenings.
- Don't stew in misery if you have tried to sleep for 20 minutes without success. Get up and stretch or read a book until you become drowsy.

NOTEBOOK ACTIVITY: TRACK YOUR SLEEP

Document your sleep and wake times for one week. It is ok to approximate this. If you note that you are not getting proper sleep, try some of the sleep hygiene tips and see if they make a difference. Keep track of what you discover in your notebook.

CONCLUSION

"Be not afraid of growing slowly; be afraid only of standing still."
~ Chinese Proverb

You have officially completed this 30-day voyage, but your travels have just begun. Go back through your notebook and review your progress. Share your experiences with a friend. Hone the skills you learned and apply them regularly in daily life. Teach them to others. You have joined the ranks of aging heroes and now have an obligation to make the world a better place by modeling a vibrant life of purpose and meaning.

Once, a Zen Master acknowledged that a student monk had achieved enlightenment. The other monks asked their newly enlightened brother what it felt like. He replied, "I'm as miserable as ever!" Enlightenment is not a final product. It is the process of constantly striving to improve and develop. The greatest heroes are fallible. We are not aging heroes because we never fail but because we keep trying despite our failures. Rough seas are part of the passage.

Life is not a perfect science. There are lots of moving parts. At first, balanced development for all of life's domains can be like spinning plates. You have to be tuned in to what area needs your attention at any given moment. In time, moving from one area to the next should be a natural part of living and should happen with little or no effort. Achieving this takes a little practice, but once you have it, you have it. When you first learned to tie your shoes as a child, the task took great concentration. Eventually, shoe tying became natural and automatic. The same is true for personal development. Once you get the fire lit, it will burn without much help from you.

Sometimes, being an aging hero may draw the attention of people close to you. Some of them will notice the changes in you and admire your courage. Others may not like the new you because you have broken away from your assigned roles. Regardless, what matters is how you see yourself. Take pride in who you are, and stand tall. What you are doing is important. The changes you make create positive ripples in the social fabric. In a very real way, your development will change the world for the better. Holism.

REFERENCES

[i] H. Jackson Brown Jr., & Internet Archive. (1991). P.S. I Love You. In *Internet Archive*. Thomas Nelson. https://archive.org/details/psiloveyou00hjac

[ii] *Regrets of the Dying*. (2018, January 7). Bronnie Ware. https://bronnieware.com/blog/regrets-of-the-dying/

[iii] *"As You Are": What the World Can Learn From Desmond Tutu*. (2012, December 20). HuffPost UK. https://www.huffingtonpost.co.uk/sophie-turton/as-you-are-what-the-world-can-learn_b_2337742.html

[iv] Dinesen, I., & Internet Archive. (1934). Seven Gothic tales. In *Internet Archive*. New York : H. Smith and R. Haas. https://archive.org/details/sevengothictales0000dine

[v] Kruse, K. (n.d.). *Zig Ziglar: 10 Quotes That Can Change Your Life*. Forbes. Retrieved February 22, 2022, from https://www.forbes.com/sites/kevinkruse/2012/11/28/zig-ziglar-10-quotes-that-can-change-your-life/?sh=6808a6c526a0

[vi] *Complete Poems: Amazon.co.uk: Emily Dickinson, Thomas H Johnson: 8601300332567: Books*. (2021). Amazon.co.uk. https://www.amazon.co.uk/gp/product/0571108644/ref=as_li_tl?ie=UTF8&camp=1634&creative=6738&creativeASIN=0571108644&linkCode=as2&tag=intereslitera-21

[vii] Orenstein, Gabriel, and Lindsay Lewis. "Erikson's Stages of Psychosocial Development." *The National Center for Biotechnology Information*, Bookshelf, 14 Nov. 2021, https://www.ncbi.nlm.nih.gov/books/NBK556096/.

viii "Money Buys Happiness When You Spend On Others, Study Shows." *Science Daily*, Science Daily, 21 Mar. 2008, https://www.sciencedaily.com/releases/2008/03/080320150034.htm.

ix Carter, Sherrie. "Helper's High: The Benefits (and Risks) of Altruism | Psychology Today." *Psychology Today*, Psychology Today, 4 Sept. 2014, https://www.psychologytoday.com/us/blog/high-octane-women/201409/helpers-high-the-benefits-and-risks-altruism.

x Wood, Graeme. "Secret Fears of the Super-Rich - The Atlantic." *The Atlantic*, https://www.facebook.com/TheAtlantic/, 24 Feb. 2011, https://www.theatlantic.com/magazine/archive/2011/04/secret-fears-of-the-super-rich/308419/.

xi Luthar, Suniya, and Shawn Latendresse. "Children of the Affluent." *PubMed Central (PMC)*, Curr Dir Psychol Sci, 14 Feb. 2005, https://www.ncbi.nlm.nih.gov/pmc/articles/PMC1948879/.

xii Orenstein, Gabriel A. "Eriksons Stages of Psychosocial Development - StatPearls - NCBI Bookshelf." *National Center for Biotechnology Information*, National Center for Biotechnology Information, 14 Nov. 2021, https://www.ncbi.nlm.nih.gov/books/NBK556096/.

xiii Mcleod, Saul. "Erik Erikson | Psychosocial Stages | Simply Psychology." *Study Guides for Psychology Students - Simply Psychology*, Simply Psychology, 2018, https://www.simplypsychology.org/Erik-Erikson.html.

xiv Fyodor Dostoyevsky. (2012). *The Double*. Dover Publications. https://www.goodreads.com/book/show/210190.The_Double

xv Petrow, S. (2018, May 24). The Gift of a Box Full of Darkness. *The New York Times*. https://www.nytimes.com/2018/05/24/well/gifts-gratitude-friendship-loss-grief-stress-poetry.html

xvi Blow, C. M. (2012, September 19). *I Know Why the Caged Bird Shrieks*. Campaign Stops. https://campaignstops.blogs.nytimes.com/2012/09/19/blow-i-know-why-the-caged-bird-shrieks/

xvii Wheeler, Michael. "Martin Heidegger (Stanford Encyclopedia of Philosophy)." *Stanford Encyclopedia of Philosophy*, 12 Oct. 2011, https://plato.stanford.edu/entries/heidegger/.

xviii "Freedom, Responsibility, and Agency – Existential Therapy." *Existential Therapy – An Introduction to Existential-Humanistic Psychology and Therapy*, 2004, https://existential-therapy.com/freedom-responsibility-and-agency/.

xix *It is not in the pursuit of happiness that we find fulfillment, it is in the happiness of pursuit.* (n.d.). Internetpoem.com. Retrieved March 1, 2022, from https://internetpoem.com/denis-waitley/quotes/it-is-not-in-the-pursuit-of-happiness-that-we-find-43040/

xx "Education Improves Decision-Making Ability, Study Finds." *Science Daily*, Science Daily, 15 Oct. 2018, https://www.sciencedaily.com/releases/2018/10/181005111436.htm.

xxi Wang, Wendy. "The Link between a College Education and a Lasting Marriage | Pew Research Center." *Pew Research Center*, https://www.facebook.com/pewresearch, 4 Dec. 2015, https://www.pewresearch.org/fact-tank/2015/12/04/education-and-marriage/.

xxii Raghupathi, Viju, and Wullianallur Raghupathi. "The Influence of Education on Health: An Empirical Assessment of OECD Countries for the Period 1995– 2015 | Archives of Public Health | Full Text." *BioMed Central*, Arch Public Health, 2020, https://archpublichealth.biomedcentral.com/articles/10.1186/s13690-020-00402-5.

xxiii quotespedia.org. (n.d.). *A gem cannot be polished without friction, nor a man perfected… – Quotespedia.org.* Www.quotespedia.org. https://www.quotespedia.org/authors/l/lucius-annaeus-seneca/a-gem-cannot-be-polished-without-friction-nor-a-man-perfected-without-trials-lucius-annaeus-seneca/

xxiv Oppong, Thomas. "Good Social Relationships Are The Most Consistent Predictor of a Happy Life." *Thrive Global: Behavior Change Platform Reducing Employee Stress and Burnout, Enhancing Performance and Well-Being*, Thrive Global, 18 Oct. 2019, https://thriveglobal.com/stories/relationships-happiness-well-being-life-lessons/.

xxv Bettina, Wiese. "Successful Pursuit of Personal Goals and Subjective Well-Being." *APA PsycNet*, APA, 2007, https://psycnet.apa.org/record/2006-11798-011.

xxvi Stephen, Post. "Altruism, Happiness, and Health: It's Good to Be Good - PubMed." *PubMed*, International Journal of Behavioral Medicine , 2005, https://pubmed.ncbi.nlm.nih.gov/15901215/.

xxvii Altorf, Marije. "Iris Murdoch and the Art of Imaging | Reviews | Notre Dame Philosophical Reviews | University of Notre Dame." *Notre Dame Philosophical Reviews*, 24 June 2009, https://ndpr.nd.edu/reviews/iris-murdoch-and-the-art-of-imaging/.

xxviii *Amazon.com: Meditations (Dover Thrift Editions) (8601420632387): Marcus Aurelius: Books*. (2000). Amazon.com. https://www.amazon.com/Meditations-Thrift-Editions-Marcus-Aurelius/dp/048629823X

xxix Noble, B. &. (n.d.). *100 Selected Poems|Paperback*. Barnes & Noble. Retrieved February 22, 2022, from https://www.barnesandnoble.com/w/100-selected-poems-e-e-cummings/1013352507

xxx *Sitting Bull: "The warrior is not someone who fights."* (2018, August 19). Historical Snapshots. https://historicalsnaps.com/2018/08/19/sitting-bull-the-warrior-is-not-someone-who-fights/

xxxi Nin, Anais, and Gunther Stuhlmann. *The Diary of Anais Nin: Vol. 3*. New York: Harcourt Brace Jovanovich, 1969. Print.

xxxii *REL2-38VM: The Art of War - Sun Tzu - Oxford University Press : Free Download, Borrow, and Streaming*. (n.d.). Internet Archive. Retrieved February 22, 2022, from https://archive.org/details/perma_cc_REL2-38VM

xxxiii *A quote by Confucius.* (n.d.). Www.goodreads.com. Retrieved March 9, 2022, from https://www.goodreads.com/quotes/8688305-the-man-who-chases-two-rabbits-catches-neither

xxxiv Migliore, Loren. "I Can't Decide! Why An Increase in Choices Decreases Our Happiness » Brain World." *Brain World,* https://www.facebook.com/brainworldmagazine/, 7 Dec. 2019, https://brainworldmagazine.com/cant-decide-increase-choices-decreases-happiness/.

xxxv *Jeanette Coron Quotes (Author of Destined for Greatness) (page 4 of 5).* (n.d.). Www.goodreads.com. Retrieved February 22, 2022, from https://www.goodreads.com/author/quotes/7704861.Jeanette_Coron?page=4

xxxvi Daniel, David, et al. "Why Cognitive Behavioral Therapy Is the Current Gold Standard of Psychotherapy." *PubMed Central (PMC),* Frontiers in Psychiatry, 29 Jan. 2018, https://www.ncbi.nlm.nih.gov/pmc/articles/PMC5797481/.

xxxvii Karlsson, Hasse. "How Psychotherapy Changes the Brain." *Psychiatric Times,* Psychiatric Times, 12 Aug. 2011, https://www.psychiatrictimes.com/view/how-psychotherapy-changes-brain.

xxxviii *Oprah's secret 1992 racism experiment on her audience is still incredible today.* (2019, September 13). Upworthy. https://www.upworthy.com/oprah-blue-eyes-brown-eyes--racism-experiment

xxxix *Why, Exactly, Is Knowing Half the Battle?* (2020, August 1). MEL Magazine. https://melmagazine.com/en-us/story/why-exactly-is-knowing-half-the-battle

xl Owen, S. (2016). 500 Relationships and life quotes: bite-sized advice for busy people. In *Open WorldCat.* https://www.worldcat.org/title/500-relationships-and-life-quotes-bite-sized-advice-for-busy-people/oclc/966309357&referer=brief_results

xli *The Quotations Page: Quote from Pythagoras.* (n.d.). The Quotations Page. Retrieved March 9, 2022, from http://www.quotationspage.com/quote/29155.html

xlii Butler, N. M. (1951). Commencement addresses; In *Open WorldCat.* Shurtleff College Press. https://www.worldcat.org/title/commencement-addresses/oclc/3051138

xliii Rozanski, Alan, et al. "Association of Optimism With Cardiovascular Events and All-Cause Mortality: A Systematic Review and Meta-Analysis | Cardiology | JAMA Network Open | JAMA Network." *JAMA Network | Home of JAMA and the Specialty Journals of the American Medical Association*, JAMA Network, 27 Sept. 2019, https://jamanetwork.com/journals/jamanetworkopen/fullarticle/2752100.

xliv Lear, Scott. "How Optimism Benefits Your Health | Heart and Stroke Foundation." *Heart and Stroke Foundation of Canada*, 5 Mar. 2020, https://www.heartandstroke.ca/articles/how-optimism-benefits-your-health.

xlv Hernandez, Rosalba, et al. "Optimism and Cardiovascular Health: Multi-Ethnic Study of Atherosclerosis (MESA)." *PubMed Central (PMC)*, Health Behav Policy Rev, 1 Jan. 2015, https://www.ncbi.nlm.nih.gov/pmc/articles/PMC4509598/.

xlvi Kim, Eric, et al. "Optimism and Cause-Specific Mortality: A Prospective Cohort Study | American Journal of Epidemiology | Oxford Academic." *OUP Academic*, Oxford University Press, 4 Jan. 2017, https://academic.oup.com/aje/article/185/1/21/2631298?login=false.

xlvii Deborah, Danner, et al. "Positive Emotions in Early Life and Longevity: Findings from the Nun Study." *APA*, Journal of Personality and Social Psychology, 2001, https://www.apa.org/pubs/journals/releases/psp805804.pdf.

xlviii Vaish, Amrisha et al. "Not All Emotions Are Created Equal: The Negativity Bias in Social-Emotional Development." *PubMed Central (PMC)*, 13 May 2013, https://www.ncbi.nlm.nih.gov/pmc/articles/PMC3652533/.

[xlix] Cookson, G. M. (n.d.). Goethe Faust. In *Internet Archive*. George Routledge and Sons Ltd., London. Retrieved February 22, 2022, from https://archive.org/details/dli.ministry.02346/page/19/mode/2up

[l] *Are you happier in your 40s or 80s? Age and happiness.* (2017, March 8). NW Health Blog. https://wa-health.kaiserpermanente.org/whos-happier-people-in-their-40s-or-80s/

[li] Williamson, M. (1994). Illuminata: Thoughts, Prayers, Rites of Passage. In *Google Books*. Random House. https://books.google.com/books?id=-Wob7DWqFJ8C&pg=PA7&lpg=PA7&dq=personal+transformation+can+and+does+have+global+effects.+As+we+go

[lii] Sapolsky, R. M. (1982). The endocrine stress-response and social status in the wild baboon. *Hormones and Behavior*, *16*(3), 279–292. https://doi.org/10.1016/0018-506x(82)90027-7

[liii] Payne, K. (n.d.). *The Myth of Executive Stress*. Scientific American. https://www.scientificamerican.com/article/the-myth-of-executive-str/

[liv] R. Morgan Griffin. (2010, May 11). *10 Health Problems Related to Stress That You Can Fix*. WebMD; WebMD. https://www.webmd.com/balance/stress-management/features/10-fixable-stress-related-health-problems

[lv] Crum, A. J., Salovey, P., & Achor, S. (2013). Rethinking stress: The role of mindsets in determining the stress response. *Journal of Personality and Social Psychology*, *104*(4), 716–733. https://doi.org/10.1037/a0031201

[lvi] *Quotes about Intellectual Growth (27 quotes)*. (n.d.). Www.quotemaster.org. Retrieved March 7, 2022, from https://www.quotemaster.org/Intellectual+Growth

[lvii] Brown, R. E. (2016). Hebb and Cattell: The Genesis of the Theory of Fluid and Crystallized Intelligence. *Frontiers in Human Neuroscience*, *10*. https://doi.org/10.3389/fnhum.2016.00606

[lviii] Joseph, Ebenezer et al. "Chess Training Improves Cognition in Children." *Research Gate*, Journal of Psychology , 2016, https://www.researchgate.net/publication/327337702_Chess_training_improves_cognition_in_children.

[lix] Preidt, Robert. "Sudoku, Crosswords Could Make Your Brain Years Younger." *MedicineNet*, MedicineNet, 16 May 2019, https://www.medicinenet.com/script/main/art.asp?articlekey=221074.

[lx] Fissler, Patrick et al. "Jigsaw Puzzling Taps Multiple Cognitive Abilities and Is a Potential Protective Factor for Cognitive Aging." *PubMed Central (PMC)*, Fronteirs in Aging Neuroscience, 1 Oct. 2018, https://www.ncbi.nlm.nih.gov/pmc/articles/PMC6174231/.

[lxi] Jarvis, Michael. "Meditation Improves Cognition, Studies Show | American Association for the Advancement of Science." *American Association for the Advancement of Science*, 4 Oct. 2017, https://www.aaas.org/news/meditation-improves-cognition-studies-show.

[lxii] Anderer, John. "Bilingual Benefits: Learning a Second Language Boosts Brain Health - Study Finds." *Study Finds*, https://www.facebook.com/StudyFindsorg/, 28 Oct. 2021, https://www.studyfinds.org/learning-second-language-brain/.

[lxiii] Schellenberg, Glen. "Music Lessons Enhance IQ." *Sage Journals*, 1 Aug. 2004, https://journals.sagepub.com/doi/abs/10.1111/j.0956-7976.2004.00711.x.

[lxiv] Conyers, Marcus, and Donna Wilson. "Smart Moves: Powering up the Brain with Physical Activity." *Sage Jounals*, 20 Apr. 2015, https://journals.sagepub.com/doi/abs/10.1177/0031721715583961.

[lxv] Hurley, Dan. "Can Reading Make You Smarter? | Books | The Guardian." *The Guardian*, The Guardian, 23 Jan. 2014, https://www.theguardian.com/books/2014/jan/23/can-reading-make-you-smarter.

[lxvi] "Critical Thinking Definition & Meaning | Dictionary.Com." *Www.Dictionary.Com*, https://www.dictionary.com/browse/critical-thinking. Accessed 24 Jan. 2022.

lxvii Makowsky, V. (2013). Editor's Introduction: New Perspectives on Puerto Rican, Latina/o, Chicana/o, and Caribbean American Literatures. *MELUS: Multi-Ethnic Literature of the United States, 38*(2), 1–4. https://doi.org/10.1093/melus/mlt021

lxviii Breen, R. G. (1964). With Mencken Memorabilia. *The Baltimore Sun*, p. 15. https://en.wikiquote.org/wiki/H._L._Mencken#A_Book_of_Prefaces_(1917)

lxx *3-2-1: How to rebound from a mistake and think outside your constraints.* (n.d.). James Clear. Retrieved March 9, 2022, from https://jamesclear.com/3-2-1/june-10-2021

lxxi Kruger, J., and D. Dunning. "Unskilled and Unaware of It: How Difficulties in Recognizing One's Own Incompetence Lead to Inflated Self-Assessments - PubMed." *PubMed*, Semantic Scholar, 30 Nov. 1999, https://pubmed.ncbi.nlm.nih.gov/10626367/.

lxxii *Bertrand Russell : The Triumph of Stupidity.* (n.d.). Russell-J.com. Retrieved March 9, 2022, from https://russell-j.com/0583TS.HT

lxxiii *thedescentofman02300gut directory listing.* (n.d.). Archive.org. Retrieved March 9, 2022, from https://archive.org/download/thedescentofman02300gut

lxxiv S, P. (2014, September 15). *Oprah Winfrey on Career, Life and Leadership (Transcript).* The Singju Post. https://singjupost.com/oprah-winfrey-career-life-leadership-transcript/

lxxv *Spirituality: A Brief History, 2nd Edition | Wiley.* (n.d.). Wiley.com. Retrieved February 22, 2022, from https://www.wiley.com/en-us/Spirituality%3A+A+Brief+History%2C+2nd+Edition-p-9781118472354

lxxvi Henderson, J. (n.d.). *On Listening to Lectures.* Loeb Classical Library. Retrieved February 22, 2022, from https://www.loebclassics.com/view/plutarch-moralia_listening_lectures/1927/pb_LCL197.201.xml [lxxvii] Gagnon, Steve. "Questions and Answers - How Much of an Atom Is Empty Space?" *Science Education at Jefferson Lab*, https://education.jlab.org/qa/how-much-of-an-atom-is-empty-space.html#:~:text=A%20hydrogen%20atom%20is%20about,the%20size%20of%20the%20earth. Accessed 25 Jan. 2022.

[lxxviii] Habe, Katarina, and et al. "Flow and Satisfaction With Life in Elite Musicians and Top Athletes." *PubMed Central (PMC)*, Frontiers in Psychology, 29 Mar. 2019, https://www.ncbi.nlm.nih.gov/pmc/articles/PMC6450199/.

[lxxix] Rawls, J. (2001). *Justice as fairness : a restatement.* (E. Kelly, Ed.). Bleknap Press Of Havard University Press.

[lxxx] Schoolzine, & Schoolzine. (n.d.). *Emmanuel College Warrnambool eNewsletter*. Emmanuel College Warrnambool ENewsletter. Retrieved February 22, 2022, from https://emmanuelcw.schoolzineplus.com/enews?nid=17

[lxxxi] Stoppler, Melissa. "Meditation, Stress, and Your Health." *WebMD*, WebMD, 28 July 2020, https://www.webmd.com/balance/guide/meditation-natural-remedy-for-insomnia#1.

[lxxxii] Newberg, Andrew, and et al. "Meditation Effects on Cognitive Function and Cerebral Blood Flow In Subjects with Memory Loss: A Preliminary Study." *Google Scholar*, Journal of Alzheimer's Disease, 12 Jan. 2010, http://scholar.google.com/scholar_url?url=http://www.andrewnewberg.com/s/meditation-effects-on-cognitive-function-and-cerebral-blood-flow-in-subjects-with-memory-loss-a-prel.pdf&hl=en&sa=X&scisig=AAGBfm1va2VwoTGJtPJdSJ71AgOxmwTgIw&nossl=1&oi=scholarr.

[lxxxiii] Spadaro, Kathleen, and et al. "Effect of Mindfulness Meditation on Short-Term Weight Loss and Eating Behaviors in Overweight and Obese Adults: A Randomized Controlled Trial - PubMed." *PubMed*, J Complement Integr Med ., 5 Dec. 2017, https://pubmed.ncbi.nlm.nih.gov/29211681/.

[lxxxiv] Szalavitz, Maia. "Explaining Why Meditators May Live Longer | TIME.Com." *TIME.Com*, https://www.facebook.com/TIMEHealthland, 23 Dec.

2010, https://healthland.time.com/2010/12/23/could-meditation-extend-life-intriguing-possibility-raised-by-new-study/.

lxxxv *The Best Buddhist Writing 2007: McLeod, Melvin: 9781590304976: Amazon.com: Books.* (2021). Amazon.com. https://www.amazon.com/Best-Buddhist-Writing-2007/dp/1590304977#:~:text=The%20Best%20Buddhist%20Writing%202007%20Paperback%20E2%80%93%20October%209%2C%202007&text=Selected%20by%20the%20editors%20of

lxxxvi Kang, Do-Hyung, and et al. "The Effect of Meditation on Brain Structure: Cortical Thickness Mapping and Diffusion Tensor Imaging." *PubMed Central (PMC)*, Soc Cogn Affect Neurosci., 8 June 2012, https://www.ncbi.nlm.nih.gov/pmc/articles/PMC3541490/.

lxxxvii *Thich Nhat Hanh on life, war and happiness • USMAIL24.* (2022, January 22). USMAIL24. https://usmail24.com/thich-nhat-hanh-on-life-war-and-happiness/

lxxxviii Hoffman, E. H., & Hoffman, C. D. (2006). Staying Focused in the Age of Distraction: How Mindfulness, Prayer and Meditation Can Help You Pay Attention to What Really Matters. In *Google Books.* New Harbinger Publications.

lxxxix *The Ultimate Book of Quotations: Demakis, Joseph M: 9781481053020: Amazon.com: Books.* (2021). Amazon.com. https://www.amazon.com/Ultimate-Book-Quotations-Joseph-Demakis/dp/1481053027

xc OpenLibrary.org. (n.d.). *Walden and Civil Disobedience (2006 edition) | Open Library.* Open Library. Retrieved February 28, 2022, from https://openlibrary.org/works/OL55649W/Walden?edition=ia%3Acu31924021445741

xci Chicago. Hopper, Dennis. 1969. Easy Rider. United States: Columbia Pictures.

xcii U.S. Dept. of Justice, *Motorcycle Gangs*, archived from the original on 2014-04-15, retrieved 2020-11-22 [xciii] Friedman, William, and et al. "Aging and the Speed of Time - ScienceDirect." *ScienceDirect.Com | Science, Health and Medical Journals, Full Text Articles and Books.*, Acta Psychologica, June 2010, https://www.sciencedirect.com/science/article/abs/pii/S0001691810000132.

[xciv] Rampton, John. "7 Reasons Why Spending Money on Experiences Makes Us Happier Than Buying Stuff." *Entrepreneur*, Entrepreneur, 15 May 2017, https://www.entrepreneur.com/article/294163.

[xcv] Kumar, Amit, and et al. "Spending on Doing Promotes More Moment-to-Moment Happiness than Spending on Having - ScienceDirect." *ScienceDirect.Com | Science, Health and Medical Journals, Full Text Articles and Books.*, Journal of Experimental Social Psychology, May 2020, https://www.sciencedirect.com/science/article/abs/pii/S0022103119305256?via%3 Dihub.

[xcvi] Newton, Michael. "The Child of Nature: The Feral Child and the State of Nature." *UCL Discovery* , 1996, https://discovery.ucl.ac.uk/1317523/1/244110.pdf.

[xcvii] Fang, Zhou, and et al. "Post-Conventional Moral Reasoning Is Associated with Increased Ventral Striatal Activity at Rest and during Task | Scientific Reports." *Nature*, Springer Nature, 2 Aug. 2017, https://www.nature.com/articles/s41598-017-07115-w.

[xcviii] Dill, Russell. *LSU Digital Commons*, LSU Historical Dissertations and Theses, 1994, https://digitalcommons.lsu.edu/gradschool_disstheses/5723.

[xcix] *Day of Affirmation Address, University of Capetown, Capetown, South Africa, June 6, 1966 | JFK Library.* (n.d.). Www.jfklibrary.org. https://www.jfklibrary.org/learn/about-jfk/the-kennedy-family/robert-f-kennedy/robert-f-kennedy-speeches/day-of-affirmation-address-university-of-capetown-capetown-south-africa-june-6-1966

[c] Zinn, H. (2004). *Voices of a people's history of the United States /*. Seven Stories Press. https://adams.marmot.org/Record/.b25355302

ci *(PDF) Research on Creativity*. (n.d.). ResearchGate.
https://www.researchgate.net/publication/257946313_Research_on_Creativity

cii da Costa, Silvia, and et al. "Personal Factors of Creativity: A Second Order Meta-Analysis - ScienceDirect." *ScienceDirect.Com | Science, Health and Medical Journals, Full Text Articles and Books.*, Revista de Psicología del Trabajo y de las Organizaciones, Dec. 2015,
https://www.sciencedirect.com/science/article/pii/S1576596215000407.

ciii Baas, M., and et al. "A Meta-Analysis of 25 Years of Mood-Creativity Research: Hedonic Tone, Activation, or Regulatory Focus?" *APA PsycNet*, APA, 1 Nov. 2008, https://psycnet.apa.org/doiLanding?doi=10.1037%2Fa0012815.

civ Conner, Tamlin, and et al. "Everyday Creative Activity as a Path to Flourishing: The Journal of Positive Psychology: Vol 13, No 2." *Taylor & Francis*, Journal of Positive Psychology, 27 Jan. 2016,
https://www.tandfonline.com/doi/abs/10.1080/17439760.2016.1257049?scroll=to p&needAccess=true&journalCode=rpos20.

cv "Creativity and Academic Achievement: A Meta-Analysis." *APA PsycNet*, Journal of Educational Psychology, Feb. 2017, https://psycnet.apa.org/buy/2016-40090-001.

cvi *Think Again: The Power of Knowing What You Don't Know: Grant, Adam: 9781984878106: Amazon.com: Books*. (2021). Amazon.com.
https://www.amazon.com/Think-Again-Power-Knowing-What/dp/1984878107

cvii *The Interpretation of Dreams*. (n.d.). Freud Museum London.
https://www.freud.org.uk/education/resources/the-interpretation-of-dreams/

cviii *3 science-based strategies to increase your creativity*. (2021, January 29). Ideas.ted.com. https://ideas.ted.com/3-science-based-strategies-to-increase-your-creativity/

cix *Courage, Compassion, and Connection: The Gifts of Imperfection.* (n.d.). Oprah.com. Retrieved February 22, 2022, from https://www.oprah.com/own-super-soul-sunday/excerpt-the-gifts-of-imperfection-by-dr-brene-brown/5

cx *The True Voice of Love.* (n.d.). Henri Nouwen. Retrieved February 22, 2022, from https://henrinouwen.org/meditations/the-true-voice-of-love/

cxi von Mohr, Mariana, and et al. "The Soothing Function of Touch: Affective Touch Reduces Feelings of Social Exclusion." *PubMed Central (PMC)*, Scientific Reports, 18 Oct. 2017, https://www.ncbi.nlm.nih.gov/pmc/articles/PMC5647341/.

cxii Keltner, Dacher. "Hands On Research: The Science of Touch." *Greater Good*, Greater Good Magazine, 29 Sept. 2010, https://greatergood.berkeley.edu/article/item/hands_on_research.

cxiii Keltner, Dacher. "Hands On Research: The Science of Touch." *Greater Good*, Greater Good Magazine, 29 Sept. 2010, https://greatergood.berkeley.edu/article/item/hands_on_research.

cxiv Holland, Kimberly. "Intimacy vs Isolation: The Importance of Relationships in Adulthood." *Healthline*, Healthline Media, 8 July 2019, https://www.healthline.com/health/mental-health/intimacy-vs-isolation.

cxv Fehr, B. "Self-Disclosure - an Overview | ScienceDirect Topics." *ScienceDirect.Com | Science, Health and Medical Journals, Full Text Articles and Books.*, Encyclopedia of Human Behavior , 2012, https://www.sciencedirect.com/topics/psychology/self-disclosure.

cxvi Jourard, S. M. (1971). The Transparent Self. In *Google Books*. Van Nostrand Reinhold. https://www.google.com/books/edition/The_Transparent_Self/G7VPh-blX8AC?hl=en&gbpv=1&bsq=cite+original+source+jourard+1971+It+is+through+self-disclosure+that+an+individual+reveals+to+himself+and+to+the+other+party+just+ex-actly+who

cxvii DeFelice, R. (2019, June 14). *Sonya Deville: "Don't Ever Apologize for Your Sexuality, Just be You."* EWrestlingNews.com. https://www.ewrestlingnews.com/news/sonya-deville-dont-ever-apologize-for-your-sexuality-just-be-you

cxviii Robinson, Kara Mayer. "10 Surprising Health Benefits of Sex." *WebMD*, WebMD, 24 Oct. 2013, https://www.webmd.com/sex-relationships/guide/sex-and-health.

cxix Dyble, M., and et al. "Human Behavior. Sex Equality Can Explain the Unique Social Structure of Hunter-Gatherer Bands - PubMed." *PubMed*, National Library of Medicine, 15 May 2015, https://pubmed.ncbi.nlm.nih.gov/25977551/.

cxx Keltner, Dacher. "Hands On Research: The Science of Touch." *Greater Good*, Greater Good Magazine, 29 Sept. 2010, https://greatergood.berkeley.edu/article/item/hands_on_research.

cxxi McCool, M., and et al. "Thieme E-Journals - Das Gesundheitswesen / Abstract." *Home - Thieme Connect*, Das Gesundheitswesen, 2015, https://www.thieme-connect.com/products/ejournals/abstract/10.1055/s-0035-1563097.

cxxii Cowden, Craig, and et al. "Religiosity and Sexual Concerns: International Journal of Sexual Health: Vol 19, No 1." *Taylor & Francis*, International Journal of Sexual Health, 29 Apr. 2005, https://www.tandfonline.com/doi/abs/10.1300/J514v19n01_03.

cxxiii *News & Notes – 21st Century Chaplains Network.* (n.d.). https://21ccn.org/news-notes/

cxxiv Holt-Lunstad, Julianne, et al. "(PDF) Loneliness and Social Isolation as Risk Factors for Mortality: A Meta-Analytic Review." *ResearchGate*, Perspectives on Psychological Science, 11 Mar. 2015, https://www.researchgate.net/publication/273910450_Loneliness_and_Social_Isolation_as_Risk_Factors_for_Mortality_A_Meta-Analytic_Review.

cxxv Field, Tiffany, and et al. "Preterm Infant Massage Therapy Research: A Review." *PubMed Central (PMC)*, Infant Behav Dev, Apr. 2010, https://www.ncbi.nlm.nih.gov/pmc/articles/PMC2844909/.

cxxvi Markman, Art. "Why Other People Are the Key to Our Happiness | Psychology Today." *Psychology Today*, Psychology Today, 22 July 2014, https://www.psychologytoday.com/us/blog/ulterior-motives/201407/why-other-people-are-the-key-our-happiness?fbclid=IwAR3khRAsIjCBVgNvF5qhWsdWkVWUFYkukPaYLKJeNxxBIxYiBmm9qNNaRvM.

cxxvii May, R. (2009). *Man's search for himself.* Norton.

cxxviii *Yves Saint Laurent, Style is Eternal.* (n.d.). Musée Yves Saint Laurent Paris. Retrieved March 9, 2022, from https://museeyslparis.com/en/international-exhibitions/yves-saint-laurent-style-is-eternal#:~:text=%E2%80%9CFashion%20fades%2C%20style%20is%20eternal

cxxix *Psychotherapy East and West: Watts, Alan W.: 9780394716091: Amazon.com: Books.* (2021). Amazon.com. https://www.amazon.com/Psychotherapy-East-West-Alan-Watts/dp/0394716094

cxxx Crammer, Phebe. "Identity, Narcissism, and Defense Mechanisms in Late Adolescence." *APA PsycNet*, Journal of Research in Personality, 1995, https://psycnet.apa.org/record/1996-10949-001.

cxxxi *StackPath.* (n.d.). Movemequotes.com. https://movemequotes.com/health-and-fitness-quotes/

cxxxii Festini, Sara, and et al. "The Busier the Better: Greater Busyness Is Associated with Better Cognition." *PubMed Central (PMC)*, Front Aging Neurosci, 2016, https://www.ncbi.nlm.nih.gov/pmc/articles/PMC4870334/.

cxxxiii "Ernestine Shepherd Workout Routine and Diet Plan." *Fitness Clone*, https://www.facebook.com/fitnessclone/, 15 July 2019, https://fitnessclone.com/ernestine-shepherd-workout-diet/.

cxxxiv "Carrie Johnson." *Team USA*, Team USA, https://www.teamusa.org/Athletes/JO/Carrie-Johnson.aspx. Accessed 25 Jan. 2022.

cxxxv "Scott Hamilton Quotes - BrainyQuote." *BrainyQuote*, https://www.brainyquote.com/authors/scott-hamilton-quotes. Accessed 25 Jan. 2022.

cxxxvi Ladd, Madeline. "Just Keep Swimming: 5 Ways to Overcome a Plateau." *Swimming World News*, https://www.facebook.com/SwimmingWorld, 21 Oct. 2021, https://www.swimmingworldmagazine.com/news/just-keep-swimming-5-ways-to-overcome-a-plateau/#:~:text=%E2%80%9CIt's%20what%20you%20do%20with,be%20able%20to%20break%20through.

cxxxvii *The best training program in the world is absolutely worthless without the will to execute it properly, consistently, and with intensity. - John Romaniello*. (n.d.). Www.allgreatquotes.com. Retrieved February 22, 2022, from https://www.allgreatquotes.com/quote-241987/

cxxxviii "Fitness Training: Elements of a Well-Rounded Routine - Mayo Clinic." *Mayo Clinic*, Mayo Clinic, 22 Sept. 2020, https://www.mayoclinic.org/healthy-lifestyle/fitness/in-depth/fitness-training/art-20044792.

cxxxix "Preserve Your Muscle Mass - Harvard Health." *Harvard Health*, 19 Feb. 2016, https://www.health.harvard.edu/staying-healthy/preserve-your-muscle-mass.

cxl Swartzendruber, Kris. "Strength Training Offers Many Health Benefits - MSU Extension." *MSU Extension*, Michigan State University, 9 Oct. 2012, https://www.canr.msu.edu/news/strength_training_offers_many_health_benefits#:~:text=Strength%20training%20may%20also%20help,Parkinson's%20disease%2C%20arthritis%20and%20fibromyalgia.

cxli Willis, Leslie, and et al. "Effects of Aerobic and/or Resistance Training on Body Mass and Fat Mass in Overweight or Obese Adults - PubMed." *PubMed*, J Appl Physiol , 27 Sept. 2012, https://pubmed.ncbi.nlm.nih.gov/23019316/.

cxlii Steel, James, and et al. "Long-Term Time-Course of Strength Adaptation to Minimal Dose Resistance Training: Retrospective Longitudinal Growth Modeling of a Large Cohort through Training Records." *ResearchGate*, Jan. 2021, https://www.researchgate.net/publication/348824509_Long-term_time-course_of_strength_adaptation_to_minimal_dose_resistance_training_Retrospective_longitudinal_growth_modelling_of_a_large_cohort_through_training_records.

cxliii *Captain Jacked: Zach McGowan's Black Sails Workout.* (2014, January 27). Muscle & Fitness. https://www.muscleandfitness.com/workouts/athletecelebrity-workouts/captain-jacked-zach-mcgowans-black-sails-workout/

cxliv "How Many Total Sets Should I Do during My Strength Training? | Strength Training & Exercise - Sharecare." *Sharecare*, National Academy of Sports Medicine, https://www.sharecare.com/health/strength-training/sets-during-strength-training. Accessed 25 Jan. 2022.

cxlv Kato, Michitaka, and et al. "IJERPH | Free Full-Text | The Efficacy of Stretching Exercises on Arterial Stiffness in Middle-Aged and Older Adults: A Meta-Analysis of Randomized and Non-Randomized Controlled Trials." *MDPI*, Multidisciplinary Digital Publishing Institute, 2 Aug. 2020, https://www.mdpi.com/1660-4601/17/16/5643.

cxlvi Brennan, Dan. "Passive Range of Motion and Active Range of Motion: What's the Difference?" *WebMD*, WebMD, 25 Oct. 2021, https://www.webmd.com/fitness-exercise/difference-between-passive-range-of-motion-and-active-range-of-motion#1.

cxlvii "Impact of Static Stretching on Performance - Physiopedia." *Physiopedia*, Physiopedia, https://www.physio-pedia.com/Impact_of_Static_Stretching_on_Performance. Accessed 25 Jan. 2022.

[cxlviii] *Louis C. K. Quotes*. (n.d.). BrainyQuote. Retrieved April 21, 2022, from https://www.brainyquote.com/quotes/louis_c_k_452800

[cxlix] Liles, M. (2021, August 14). *125 Inspiring Mahatma Gandhi Quotes That'll Will Change Your Life*. Parade: Entertainment, Recipes, Health, Life, Holidays. https://parade.com/1247073/marynliles/gandhi-quotes/

[cl] Daniels, Jeff. "Sailor 'sleep Deprivation' Eyed at Senate Panel on Navy Ship Accidents." *CNBC*, CNBC, 19 Sept. 2017, https://www.cnbc.com/2017/09/19/sailor-sleep-deprivation-eyed-at-senate-panel-on-navy-ship-accidents.html.

[cli] Sampson, Stacy. "11 Effects of Sleep Deprivation on Your Body." *Healthline*, Healthline Media, 15 Dec. 2021, https://www.healthline.com/health/sleep-deprivation/effects-on-body.

[clii] "CDC - How Much Sleep Do I Need? - Sleep and Sleep Disorders." *Centers for Disease Control and Prevention*, CDC, 2 Mar. 2017, https://www.cdc.gov/sleep/about_sleep/how_much_sleep.html.

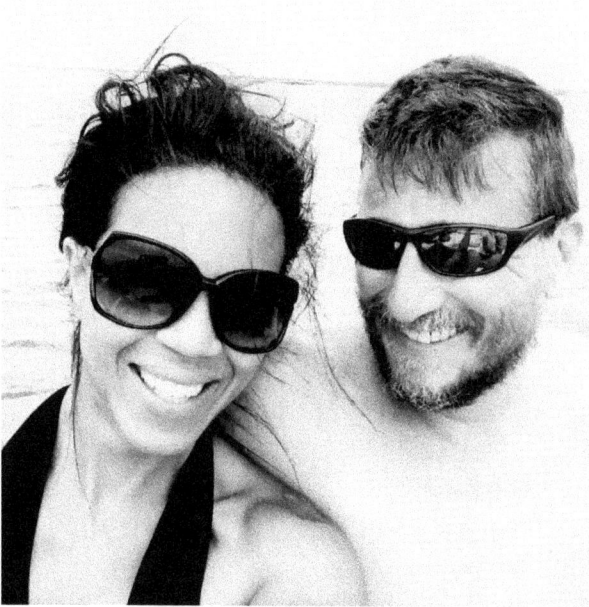

ABOUT THE AUTHORS

Randolph Harrison is a college psychology instructor, a member of the American Psychological Association, and a former counseling therapist who grew up in the sea islands of South Carolina. He received the Roston Endowed Teaching Chair and the WPCC Excellence in Teaching Award. Randolph has lectured on a wide range of psychology and education topics. Harrison is a writer, musician, motorcyclist, sailor, fitness geek, and avid outdoor adventurer.

Erica Schwarting sees life through the lens of an artist. She has a keen eye for detail and an innate talent as a designer. Schwarting manages a hospital volunteer program and spiritual care services. Being a change agent for diversity and inclusion is a value she holds dear. She is a runner who has competed in hundreds of races, including the Mt. Kilimanjaro Half-Marathon and the Chicago Marathon.

NOTE FROM THE AUTHOR

Word-of-mouth is crucial for any author to succeed. If you enjoyed *A Guide for Aging Heroes*, please leave a review online—anywhere you are able. Even if it's just a sentence or two. It would make all the difference and would be very much appreciated.

Thanks!
Randolph Harrison, MEd. and Erica Schwarting

We hope you enjoyed reading this title from:

BLACK ROSE
writing™

www.blackrosewriting.com

Subscribe to our mailing list – *The Rosevine* – and receive **FREE** books, daily deals, and stay current with news about upcoming releases and our hottest authors.
Scan the QR code below to sign up.

Already a subscriber? Please accept a sincere thank you for being a fan of Black Rose Writing authors.

View other Black Rose Writing titles at www.blackrosewriting.com/books and use promo code **PRINT** to receive a **20% discount** when purchasing.

www.ingramcontent.com/pod-product-compliance
Lightning Source LLC
Chambersburg PA
CBHW060501030426
42337CB00015B/1687